Vagus Nerve

All You Need To Know About Your Body's Natural Ability To Heal

Written by

Jason Cooper

© **Copyright 2019 - All rights reserved.**

The content contained within this book may not be reproduced, duplicated or transmitted without direct written permission from the author or the publisher.

Under no circumstances will any blame or legal responsibility be held against the publisher, or author, for any damages, reparation, or monetary loss due to the information contained within this book, either directly or indirectly.

Legal Notice:

This book is copyright protected. It is only for personal use. You cannot amend, distribute, sell, use, quote or paraphrase any part, or the content within this book, without the consent of the author or publisher.

Disclaimer Notice:

Please note the information contained within this document is for educational and entertainment purposes only. All effort has been executed to present accurate, up to date, reliable, complete information. No warranties of any kind are declared or implied. Readers acknowledge that the author is not engaging in the rendering of legal, financial, medical or professional advice. The content within this book has been derived from various sources. Please consult a licensed professional before attempting any techniques outlined in this book.

By reading this document, the reader agrees that under no circumstances is the author responsible for any losses, direct or indirect, that are incurred as a result of the use of information contained within this document, including, but not limited to, errors, omissions, or inaccuracies.

Table Of Contents

Table Of Contents...4

Introduction 9

  A Better Way Forward................................. 12

    How to Use This Book 14

Chapter 1: What is the Vagus Nerve? 16

  Physical and Emotional.............................. 17

    Historical Facts 18

    Branches... 21

    The Ventral Branch 23

    The Dorsal Branch..................................26

    Implications 30

Chapter 2: Where is the Vagus Nerve Located?...32

  The Nervous System and You 33

    The Cranial Nerves..................................34

    Social Engagement................................. 40

    Ninth and Eleventh Cranial Nerves 42

    Spinal Nerves 43

    Enteric Nervous System 45

Chapter 3: The Main Functions of the Vagus Nerve 47

    Influence..48

        Inflammation 48

        Memory 51

        Respiration..53

        Heart Function 55

        Relaxation 57

        Gut Health... 57

        Response to Stress................................ 61

Chapter 4: Diseases Associated With the Vagus Nerve and How to Prevent Them 63

    The Dorsal Vagal State 64

        Dizziness and Fainting 66

        POTS..67

        Memory Loss...70

        Depression and Anxiety 71

    The Ventral State...73

Chapter 5: Stress, Anxiety and the Vagus Nerve 78

    The Sympathetic Nervous System..............79

        Fight or Flight.. 81

- The Truth About Stress and Healing......84
- Chapter 6: Polyvagal Theory 93
  - Thermostats 94
    - Neural Pathways......................................96
    - Neuroception..100
    - Trauma and Neuroception 104
- Chapter 7: Testing Your Vagus Nerve 108
  - Basic Tests..109
    - The Three Faces 111
  - Physical and Emotional Malfunctions 115
    - Chronic Physical Symptoms...................116
    - Emotional Issues 117
    - Heart and Lung Issues 118
    - Bodily Function Disorders 118
    - Immunity Issues.....................................119
    - Behavioral Problems 121
    - Mental Issues 121
    - Miscellaneous Problems........................ 122
  - Heart Rate Variability 122
- Chapter 8: Activating the Vagus Nerve 126
  - Basic Tracking 127
    - S.E.A..128

Why S.E.A Works 131
The Neuro Fascial Release Technique 135
   Steps 136
   Technique 139
Massages for Migraines 140

Chapter 9: Natural Ways of Activating the Vagus Nerve 143
Level One 144
   The Half Salamander 146
Level Two 148
Releasing a Stiff Neck 149
Natural Lifestyle Methods 150
   Cold Therapy 151
   Deep Breathing 152
   Moving Your Mouth and Using Your Vocal Chords 153
   Intermittent Fasting 154
   Probiotics and Clean Diets 154
   Fats and Omega-3 157
   Variety 158

Chapter 10: Other Simple Exercises to Activate the Vagus Nerve 160
Twisting the Trapezius 160

- Steps 162
- Acuncture Techniques 163
  - Steps 164
  - Technique #2 167
- Conclusion 171
- References 176

Introduction

Your nervous system plays a huge role in regulating your stress and happiness levels. For a long time now, the commonly held belief has been that the autonomic nervous system largely functions in two states: relaxation and stress. This theory is so widespread that doctors and psychologists to this day prescribe treatments for stress, anxiety, and depression based on it.

The pharmaceutical industry earns billions of dollars per year thanks to the sales of medicines and drugs that seek to alleviate stress and other chronic illnesses. Despite all the studies that have been carried out and all of the research that is put into these drugs, our world seems to be more anxious and stress filled than ever. So what gives?

For starters, the traditional two state theory doesn't hold water. If stress and relaxation are the only states our brain lives in, how does one explain why we remain anxious after the cause of stress has passed? In order to understand this argument better, we need to look at how our brain reacts when a source of stress is spotted.

The brain contains an inbuilt bias which makes it supremely sensitive towards any perceived threat. This makes us very sensitive towards negative experiences, far more than the degree with which we seek out positive experiences. This negative bias causes a lot of problems but is actually essential for our survival.

Once a threat is detected from a source, our body switches into fight or flight mode. This is a heightened state of awareness where we're supremely aware of everything that is going on around us. Our heart beats faster and blood flow is directed towards our limbs to prep them in case they need to move quickly to avoid the threat. Our internal organs cooperate with this state of affairs and suspend their usual activities.

Things like the digestive and reproductive process take a back seat until the threat is in play. Adrenaline floods our system to power us in a given direction. All of this sounds great, but the fact is that our body and nervous system can sustain this for only so long before giving out. After all, living on the edge like this is not a long-term strategy.

Once the threat subsides, our bodily functions return to their normal levels, and this is the relaxation state. This is when we're functioning at a normal level and whatever thoughts we might be thinking, we're generally relaxed and not too concerned about our survival which allows us to indulge in things such as food and sex.

All of this is what the two state theory of our nervous system states, anyway. It isn't completely wrong and actually contains a lot of truth to it. Instead of calling it wrong, perhaps a better way to describe it is to say that it is incomplete.

A Better Way Forward

The weakness in the two state theory is clearly visible when we observe a person who is not in a threatening environment but exhibits all of the symptoms of being in one anyway. The inability of our brain to distinguish completely between these opposite situations and to fall out of balance when trying to evaluate them leads to a lot of problems.

Anxiety is simply the projection of our worries into the future. In other words we make up certain images that scare the living daylights out of us and these images, which are completely made up, are taken as real by the brain and it begins to think it is in a place where your survival is being threatened. So how does our nervous system really work and react?

Research has shown that a number of alternative therapies such as craniosacral therapy, visceral massage, and connective tissue release are effective in reducing stress levels. The connection between these therapies and the autonomous nervous system was explored further and finally resulted in the creation of the Polyvagal Theory.

Introduced by Dr. Stephen Porges of the University of Illinois, the theory aims to explain the mind and body connection. This is a huge oversimplification but I'm going to dive into this in far more detail later in this book, so don't worry. At the heart of Polyvagal Theory is the vagus nerve, which is the center of discussion in this book.

This nerve interacts with other bodily systems and plays an important role in parasympathetic control of the heart, lungs, and the digestive system. There are actually multiple vagus nerves but they're referred to in the singular. The various branches of this nerve (nerves) supports different evolutionary responses within us and this is why stimulation of the vagus nerve has a number of positive effects on well-being.

How to Use This Book

This book is going to take you on a detailed tour of the vagus nerve and of the Polyvagal theory in detail. We'll start off by looking at the details of the vagus nerve, its location and its main functions. There are various diseases which are caused by an improperly functioning vagus nerve and we'll look at these next. Stress and anxiety are simply two different facets of this.

Polyvagal theory is going to give you a better view of things and will help you understand the context in which everything works. We'll end by looking at some simple exercises you can carry out to stimulate your vagus nerve which will help you lower your anxiety and stress levels.

There are some natural ways to do this along with some simple exercises you can carry out. We'll look at all of this in detail. While activating your vagus nerve does require some work, it is more important that you keep an open mind. A lot of this material might seem like it contradicts popular opinion but in fact clarifies it. So with all of that being said, let's begin our journey into understanding the functions of the vagus nerve!

Chapter 1: What is the Vagus Nerve?

The vagus nerve is just one part of the Polyvagal theory I had mentioned earlier. This theory goes a long way in explaining the mind body connection that exists within us. In addition to this, the theory gives us a far clearer picture with regards to handling stress and managing our well-being.

Given that it is the central piece in polyvagal theory, it makes sense to understand what the vagus nerve is and how central it is to a lot of our bodily functions and emotional well-being. This chapter is going to take a deep look at this critical nerve and help you understand it biologically.

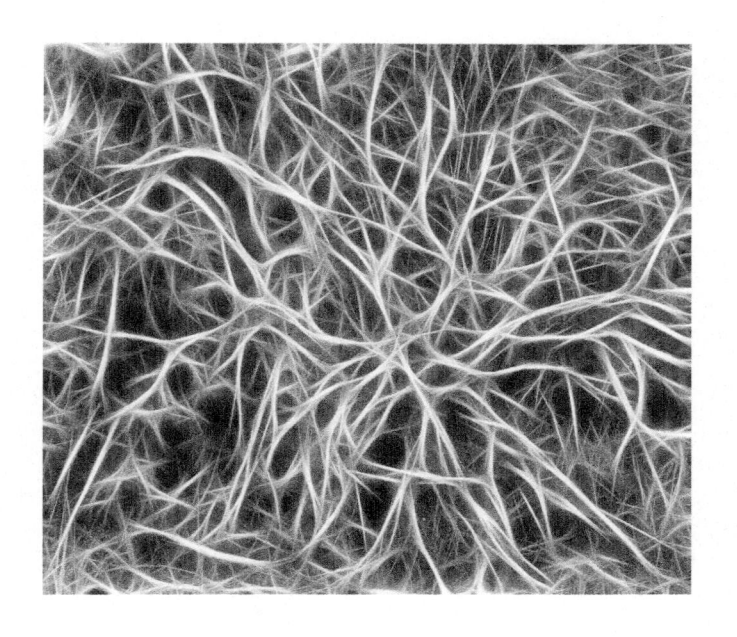

Physical and Emotional

Our mind and body are connected. How many times have you woken up after a bad night's sleep and have felt physically sluggish all day long? Also, how many times has something great happened which has caused you to feel good and all of a sudden your previous sluggishness has vanished?

The fact is that most of us know the mind and body connection intimately, but what we're not aware of is that the vagus nerve is the common thread throughout all of it. The vagus nerve is one of twelve cranial nerve pairs. Denoted as CN X biologically, this nerve travels throughout the body and transmits messages from the brain to our various organs.

Indeed, its very name 'vagus' derives from the Latin word for wandering thanks to the area it covers within us. The neck, chest, and abdomen are just some of the areas the vagus nerve wanders into and as such, a lot of our well-being is connected to it functioning well.

Historical Facts

While Polyvagal theory is a relatively new concept, the existence of the vagus nerve has long been hinted at and even experimented upon. The nervous system has long fascinated us as human beings. It is easily the most complex system in the world since not only does it combine high complexity of anatomy (which refers to the organs involved) but also physiology (which refers to the function and interaction of organs and nerves).

These days medical students spend the better half of their first few years studying both subjects in great detail. What will astonish you to learn is that a lot of the material they cover originates from ancient Rome, particularly from the works of an ancient physician named Claudius Galen who lived between 130-200 AD (Gehin, 2007). One of the reasons Galen's work is popular is due to the fact that he is one of the few people whose works have survived for so long.

Galen's primary research was conducted while treating injuries of gladiators as well as dissections of barbary apes. Galen does mention the existence of this all important nerve and physicians since then developed on his work. This led to the discovery of the fact that the nervous system was comprised of two portions: the sympathetic and parasympathetic (Gehin, 2007).

The sympathetic system boils down to the fight or flight response as detailed earlier. The parasympathetic system consists of the vagus nerve and promotes relaxation, healing and so on. This discovery is why the dual state theory came into being since researchers assumed that both systems remained in balance. If one was active, the other was inactive and so on.

The dual state theory acknowledged the importance of the vagus nerve to bodily function but only in terms of physical well-being. Given that the nerve found its way into pretty much every organ in the body, it was acknowledged that a fully functioning vagus nerve was essential for good health. In combination with a few other nerves which found their way into the gut and genitalia, the state of relaxation was thought to be simply a function of physical well-being which would be transmitted back to the brain.

Stephen Porges shook this theory to the core in 1994 when he presented a radical new concept called Polyvagal theory, which I'll cover in more detail later in this book. Porges essentially rewrote the book on the autonomic nervous system. While he agreed with the existing concept of the origin of stress, instead of focusing on two states, he focused on three divisions of the vagus nerve: the dorsal branch, the ventral branch, and the sympathetic nervous system.

Branches

Dorsal in medical terms refers to something that originates at the back, whereas ventral means originating from the front. The vagus nerve actually consists of these two branches and is technically a collection of nerves, as opposed to one single stem. The dorsal and ventral branches originate at different places in the brain and the brain stem and have different paths throughout the body.

In what is a confusing piece of trivia, these two branches don't have a whole lot to do with one another and are responsible for completely different things. So why are they both clumped together? Well, this is partly because of the original two state theory and the anatomical underpinnings of it. The vagus nerve's branches were simply combined together and there was no attempt to understand the individual roles of the branches.

Besides, nerves are complex things and it never really occurred to scientists to look at these branches for explanations until Porges came along. Not only are the branches different in function, their very structure is different. The ventral branch is myelinated, which is to say that it is covered with connective tissue cells which enable faster communication between the nerve branch and the brain.

In contrast, the dorsal branch isn't. The ventral branch has been observed to work with four other cranial nerves, namely V, VII, IX and XI, to support a range of behaviors and responses which we'll look at in a later chapter. While the sympathetic nervous system is responsible for producing the fight or flight response, both branches of the vagus nerve produce states of immobilization. Immobilization doesn't mean you'll be paralyzed, it refers to the biological functions of a person's organs and general state of mind.

However, the interesting fact to note is that the immobilization effects of both branches are very different.

The Ventral Branch

The ventral branch, in conjunction with the four cranial nerves it works with, is responsible for producing a state of calm social interaction. There are some prerequisites to healthy social interaction, namely physical health and the absence of danger or the fight or flight response. In such a state we can let our guard down and function in a state of immobility. To promote this state of well-being, the ventral branch coordinates feelings of rest and other psychological conditions which are necessary for a variety of socially important functions.

Things such as bonding with our children, forming friendships and relationships, cooperation and so on depend on the regulation of the ventral branch as a result. The ventral branch is often referred to as being the 'newer' vagus nerve branch. This has to do with how our species, and indeed everything else on this planet, evolved.

The ventral circuit is found only in mammals and is not present in any other species of vertebrates. There is some debate as to whether birds have a pathway for this but this hasn't been proved conclusive as yet (Gehin, 2007). Either way, thanks to mammals being more evolved than other vertebrates, the ventral circuit is thus referred to as being newer in terms of evolution.

When the fight or flight response takes over, the ventral circuit shuts down completely and we revert to less evolved responses such as fight or flight or withdrawal. Withdrawal can be thought of as being depression and anxiety. These primitive responses are observed quite often in creatures which do not have this circuitry within them, although withdrawal in human beings and in a reptile is a very different phenomenon (Gehin, 2007).

Contrary to existing perception, the social engagement aspect of human interaction is equally responsible for protecting us and other evolutionary responses. What I mean is that we often think of social engagement in terms of making friends and so on. However, we neglect to recognize that engaging with the world with a socially engaged attitude actually prevents us from encountering a lot of danger.

If we approach a potentially threatening situation with our fight or flight response in full swing, we'll inevitably create conflict. If we engage with it in a socially positive manner, often the potential threat diffuses itself since the other person's social engagement network activates as well. People who have healthy ventral circuits thus manage to engage their flight/fight response only as a last resort and avoid the shutdown of their socially engaged side as a result.

Once the autonomic nervous system detects a threat, it switches you from engaging in an evolved and socially engaged manner to a response akin to how a reptile views the world. If this response is inadequate as well, the brain moves into a state of shutdown and withdrawal.

The Dorsal Branch

The dorsal branch is referred to as the older Vagus nerve due to its presence in pretty much every species of vertebrates. While the ventral branch brings about a state of engagement, the dorsal branch is a little more complicated. Its essential function is to bring about a state of shutdown.

This shutdown has two kinds within it: immobilization with fear and immobilization without fear. The former refers to when our fight/flight proves to be useless, we simply give up and remain frozen. This response is brought about by fear taking us over completely. Immobilization without fear is when we're completely relaxed and the dorsal branch works in association with the ventral circuit. Think of this as choosing to be intimate with someone to form a stronger bond with them.

Given the importance of survival that every creature's biological system places on its existence, you might well wonder why would a shutdown or immobilization be a good tactic? Doesn't this open the creature to certain death? Well, immobilization can also be thought of as being a slowdown. For example, hibernation is an activity which involves the dorsal circuit.

A bear hibernating in winter is employing a survival mechanism wherein it lowers its body temperature and breathing in order to survive the tough conditions. Reptiles take this to an even greater extent by achieving near complete shutdown. This is why snakes can go on for longer periods without meals. Another example of immobilization aiding survival comes from mice.

In the face of a predator, such as a hawk, which can spot and hunt scurrying mice from miles above, a mouse completely shuts down and holds its breath, while remaining still in the face of a hawk. This makes it difficult for the hawk to spot tell tale movement which is the sign of a mouse. Once the threat passes, the mouse goes back to its usual routine.

Of course, this can backfire as well. Often, deer and mice simply freeze in the face of a predator or a threat. The phrase 'deer in the headlights' is a very apt description of a shutdown which has been prompted by fear. This is the result of an extreme shutdown where the pace of it is too quick for the creature to process what is happening.

Chronic activation of the dorsal circuit is responsible for remaining in a state of almost constant shutdown. In other words, think about how a depressed or anxious person behaves. They turn away from the world because they're unable to process everything that is going on within it. Remaining in such a state for long will lead to even higher levels of depression and anxiety.

I would like to note that when using the term depression, I'm referring to the feeling and not the medical diagnosis. This doesn't mean that a medical diagnosis of depression is somehow different. The initial feeling and diagnosis simply reflect different levels of activity in the dorsal branch, with the latter reflecting far greater activity.

Trauma or a sudden threat to our lives can lead us to shutdown completely since the survival mechanism kicks in. Of course, the reasons for this mechanism coming into action might not be justified but again, this only happens when events outside of us overtake our brain's ability to figure out what's going on. When this happens, the dorsal branch is activated as a reflex and we often end up putting ourselves in more danger.

People who can function well snap out of this state once the danger has passed but chronic activation of the dorsal circuit means that people remain in this condition for far longer than necessary.

Implications

The vagus nerve thus helps us explain states of depression or depressive moods which often appear out of nowhere. The two state theory could never explain such states since it relied on the existence of a threat to justify the fight or flight response. However, by examining the activity in both branches of the vagus nerve, we arrive at a much better explanation.

While it might not be perfect, the implications are clear. The ventral circuit often acts as a brake or as an obstacle for chronic activation of the dorsal circuit. This has enabled doctors to figure out better and less addictive treatments for depression. Also note that the dorsal circuit can equally produce feelings of depression and love.

It is the combination of the ventral circuit with the dorsal that makes all the difference. Without the ventral intervention, which activates social engagement, the dorsal branch initiates immobilization which causes depression. With the social engagement branch turned on, the dorsal branch enables us to engage in activities which are a normal part of attaining greater intimacy with another person.

Thus, both circuits are equally important for our well-being. The purpose of vagus nerve stimulation is to actually have the ventral circuit intervene with the usual activity of your dorsal circuit. If you're under a state of stress, your dorsal circuit has been activated on a chronic basis. This has made it close to impossible for you to shutdown in a healthy manner. The exercises at the end of this book will help you activate the ventral circuit within a matter of a few minutes.

Chapter 2: Where is the Vagus Nerve Located?

The vagus nerve is what is called a cranial nerve. Presenting the function and location of cranial nerves is difficult because it can be hard to avoid dense medical terms and facts. However, to understand the location and biological functions of the vagus nerve, we need to take a step back and understand the autonomous nervous system that exists within us.

This chapter is going to serve as an introduction to this topic. You will get to know your nervous system better and this will help you understand the context in which both Polyvagal theory and the vagus nerve reside.

The Nervous System and You

The nervous system is a huge entity within us and it would be impossible to describe it in full in this entire book, let alone this chapter. The nervous system is comprised of the brain, the brainstem, the cranial nerves, the spinal cord, the spinal nerves and enteric nerves.

In this chapter I'm going to focus on the autonomous nervous system which consists of the brainstem, a few cranial nerves and a few spinal nerves. The bottom line is that all of these entities have one task and one task only: to ensure your physical body survives. The vagus nerve is one of the twelve cranial nerves so let's begin by looking at these now.

The Cranial Nerves

Given the densely medical nature of this topic, I'll be simplifying a lot of the concepts and terminology within this chapter so that it can be understood easily by those unfamiliar with them. There are twelve cranial nerves which are numbered using Roman numerals. This is presumably because this is when anatomists discovered the existence of these nerves.

The nerves run from the brainstem down to the various organs within our body and are tasked with carrying messages to and fro from the brain to the organs and back. The brainstem itself exists on the underside of the brain and can be thought of as the initial portion of the spinal cord. The nerves themselves are numbered on the basis of their location.

All of the nerves begin from the base of the brain (the brainstem) and exist on either side of the brain (the base of the left and right hemispheres) in a half circle. The first nerve was named CN I by an early anatomist and every subsequent nerve was denoted using the same methodology. The individual functions of the nerves vary and in fact seem unrelated at first sight.

However, the best way to understand their function is to look at them as a whole. All the nerves are associated with your well-being and help you find food, consume it, digest it and excrete the undigested portion. Let's look at them one by one. The first nerve is denoted CN I and is referred to as the olfactory nerve.

CN I was one of the first cranial nerves to evolve within us and it has everything to do with smell. Smell is a huge factor with regards to our survival. You might dismiss it as merely judging whether someone or something smells good or not, but in earlier times, smell played an important part in helping us determine whether something was edible or not. Your reaction to various food items also beings with smell.

When a morsel of food is brought close to you, do you turn away in disgust at the smell of it or does the mere thought of it make your mouth water? If you're sexually attracted to someone, the way they smell plays an important role in arousal. Interestingly, CN I is the only nerve that has direct access to the cerebral cortex (Carney, Freedland & Veith, 2005). In other words, it transmits information directly to an older, less evolved portion of our brain without having to go through any intermediary neuron or synapse. This older portion of our brain is also responsible for forming memories and this explains why our sense of smell can help us recall old memories, whether they are good or bad.

CN II is the visual nerve and is responsible for conveying information from our retinas to our brain. The nerve transmits information to a synapse which then relays it to the occipital (back) portion of our brain for processing. Visual signals are an obvious ally to survival. Does the potential food source look nutritious or poisonous? Things such as mold and staleness can be evaluated visually.

Once something passes the visual test, we bring it closer to smell it and only then do we taste it. Our eyeballs are what we use to control our vision and take information in. CN III, CN IV and CN IX are what control these movements. These nerves are the ones that control the movement of our eyeballs in every direction. Of course, your eyeballs are not the only way in which you control your vision.

You can move your neck as well to expand the range of it. CN XI enables us to do this. While the muscles are the ones that control the physical movement, it is CN XI that transmits information to them to function in a certain way. If we don't find food or sustenance in our current spot, we turn our heads and look elsewhere.

Once you've spotted something that looks good and smells right, the next step is to ingest it to see if it tastes good. Saliva is where the digestive process begins and the mixture of food with saliva is what tells us whether something is tasty or not. CN V, CN VII and CN IX are what control the secretion of saliva. The tastier something is, the greater the amount of saliva generated so as to moisten food so that we can swallow it easily. In addition to this, saliva also initiates the digestion process by beginning the breakdown of starch (Carney, Freedland & Veith, 2005).

CN V begins the process by regulating the opening and closing of the jaw. We chew our food using our teeth and grind the food down to size. We then use CN XII to employ our tongue to move food from one side to another. CN VII enables us to relax our facial muscles and helps us use the inside of our cheeks to store food for a moment before redeploying it to either be swallowed or ground down some more. Our lips are also controlled by CN VII which are used to move food around inside our mouths.

CN VII also enables us to activate our taste buds. This, along with CN X (the vagus nerve) and CN IX, controls the way our taste buds respond to the food and transmit information back to our brain as to the integrity of said food. If it tastes fine, we swallow it. If it doesn't, we spit it out. If we decide to swallow it, we flip our tongues and into our oesophagus it goes.

Our throat muscles (CN IX) and our tongue muscles (CN XII) are the major players when it comes to swallowing, but there are other minor muscles (CN V and CN VII) which also play an important role in this. Once food reaches the stomach, CN X (the dorsal branch) helps us figure out whether we need to vomit this out or not. Of all the processes in the digestive system, swallowing is the one that involves almost all of the cranial nerves.

Outside of digestion, nerves such as CN VIII control various functions within our eardrums that helps us locate food better. In addition to this, CN V and CN VII also help us socialize better by manipulating the muscles within our auditory system. All of this is just the digestive system. There are other functions and systems which the cranial nerves are involved with as well such as determining whether we're in danger or not and relaying this information to our visceral organs. This is because switching on the fight or flight system requires these organs to cooperate and it is the cranial nerves that distribute this message.

Social Engagement

One of the most important functions of the cranial nerves is their regulation of social engagement. You've already seen how crucial the vagus nerve is to this, but the fact is that the other nerves play an important, if slightly lesser role. The most important nerves in this regard are the CN V and CN VII.

CN VII impacts several motor functions of our faces. Facial expression is an important part of communication. While all of us have the ability to change our expressions according to our will, what I'm talking about here are the smaller changes in expression that communicate interest and engagement to another person.

These involuntary tics are processed by our brains and we don't consciously realize this. CN V picks up sensory input from the skin on your face and transmits this back to your brain. Thus, CN V and VII work together to help us manipulate our facial expressions in response to social stimuli. CN VII performs another vital role with regards to our hearing.

The stapedius muscle is responsible for insulating us from our own voice. If you have a high and booming voice or if you can shriek or shout at a shrill pitch, then your own eardrum would likely suffer due to the proximity of the noise. The stapedius muscle protects the eardrum and it is CN VII which communicates information to and from it. For example, a lion contracts this muscle prior to roaring (Carney, Freedland & Veith, 2005).

On humans the stapedius muscle also allows mothers and their babies to bond. Their ears filter other sounds out and exaggerate the other's voice so a baby can hear his mother pretty well even if there are other distracting noises present. Dysfunction in these nerves often leads to symptoms such as being disturbed by the smallest of noises and so on. Tooth surgery tends to disrupt the function of one of these nerves.

Ninth and Eleventh Cranial Nerves

CN IX is responsible for a whole host of functions from swallowing to monitoring the levels of blood pressure within the body. It receives sensory information from the tongue, the tonsils and the middle ear. It also has branches in the carotid sinus which is what enables it to monitor blood pressure. Using this feedback, it manipulates the movement of the heart and muscle fibers to regulate blood pressure. It also monitors the levels of oxygen and carbon dioxide in the blood and adjusts breathing rate accordingly.

The eleventh cranial nerve CN XI is responsible for manipulation of the muscles in your back and lower neck. These affect your posture and malfunction in CN XI causes acute shoulder problems, migraines, and so on.

Spinal Nerves

The spine is one of the most important organs in our body and spinal nerves are what make communication between the brain and spine possible. Problems such as herniated discs and bone spurs on the spine can disrupt this communication. While surgical methods exist, there is a growing body of evidence that suggests that these methods might not be a good option for the long run (Gehin, 2007).

Conventional treatment methods for the spine include yoga, osteopathy, and chiropractor visits. The spinal nerve control pretty much every motor function in our body, from the movement of our limbs to the movement of our face. In addition to this, spinal nerves are also connected to our visceral organs and communicate important information back to our brain through the spinal cord.

Much like cranial nerves, there are multiple branches of spinal nerves which run within muscles. This way if a single branch fails, there is always a backup. Stress affects the proper functioning of the spinal nerves with high levels of it disabling smooth motor function. Generally speaking, when a stress response is activated, all of the spinal nerves are affected and this affects motor ability.

Under this response the spinal nerves facilitate greater explosive movement but once it subsides, the residual elements of stress often impede the body's ability to perform tasks well. Spinal nerves travel to different parts of the body and much like cranial nerves, different nerves influence the same muscle.

The nerves form what is referred to as a sympathetic chain throughout our body. Thus, when a stress response is activated by the brain, the message goes out to every portion of it. Response from our muscles is instantaneous as they prepare to spring into action. visceral organs react to this as well. The heart pumps blood in greater volume, digestion is halted as the stomach takes a back seat, and blood is rerouted towards the limbs to provide them with more oxygen.

In addition, our lungs expand as our breathing capacity increases. As you can imagine, this state of affairs doesn't last for very long and this is why a stress response causes a lot of damage. While the effects of a single response can be mitigated, continued exposure can ruin basic bodily functions since it will become so used to operating under abnormal circumstances that normal functions become abnormal.

Enteric Nervous System

The enteric nervous system is very easy to describe because we know next to nothing about it. This is often referred to as a second brain because all of its processes are automatic and we are neither conscious of it and neither can we regulate it in any way (Gehin, 2007). The enteric nerves run between the various visceral organs inside our body.

They are so tightly wound in with connective tissue that researchers cannot study or separate them to understand what their function is. It is thought that this system coordinates different internal functions between the organs. However, we don't know exactly what is being coordinated. As a result, anatomy books don't deal with these in great detail.

This brings to a close our look at the different nerves within the nervous system. As you can see, the vagus nerve is just one small cog in a much larger machine. While it is important to focus on healing and stimulating the vagus to improve your well-being, understand that your health is controlled by a number of other factors and it is unreasonable to expect one thing to cure all your ills.

In tandem with the other cranial nerves and the spinal nerves, your body has a very sophisticated system of response to stimuli. While the vagus is important, this doesn't mean the others and their functions can be ignored.

Chapter 3: The Main Functions of the Vagus Nerve

As we've seen previously, the vagus nerve is actually a combination of two different circuits. These have a number of different functions. I touched upon them briefly two chapters back but in this chapter, we're going to go on a deeper dive to understand how the nerve works and how it can help you with your stress related issues.

Again, I'll be simplifying a lot of medical terms and concepts in this chapter to help you understand the material better.

Influence

The vagus nerve affects and influences a number of different functions. These can be boiled down to the following:

- Inflammation
- Memory
- Respiration
- Heart function
- Relaxation
- Gut health
- Response to stress

Let's look at these one by one.

Inflammation

Inflammation is a normal bodily response to injury but much like stress, chronic inflammation can be harmful. Chronic pain is caused by persistent inflammation. Incidentally, fight or flight responses make the body even more susceptible to inflammation (Gehin, 2007). This is easy enough to understand why.

Your body is expecting to fall under some sort of attack and as a result preps itself to bring inflammation into the mix at the slightest provocation to mitigate the effects of any injury. Unfortunately, the body and brain cannot tell the difference between an actual threat and an imagined one. Incurring inflammation due to worrying about your job security hardly counts as a valid response.

Interestingly a healthy vagal tone, or a fully functional vagus nerve, has been found to reduce the instances of inflammation. The ventral branch in particular is what regulates the fight or flight response. By adopting a social attitude towards a situation, a person with a properly calibrated vagal tone will avoid and diffuse potential fight/flight situations before they even occur.

In addition to this, a properly functioning ventral circuit will ensure social connection, presence of relationships, and friends, which removes most of the causes of stress in life. Studies have shown that we deal with stress far better when we distribute the burden, so to speak (Gernot, 2016). A person who has social connections will fare better under stress than someone who doesn't have any to count on.

The vagus nerve's ability to regulate inflammation also extends to reducing inflammation that arises due to arthritis. Studies have shown that stimulating the vagus nerve in arthritic patients reduces inflammation thanks to increased production of cytokines (Gernot, 2016). Cytokines are effectively what prohibit inflammation and thus the vagus nerve seems to play a key role in this.

Exactly how the vagus nerve enhances the production of cytokines is not known. One possible speculation indicates that the neural circuitry which produces them is influenced by the vagus nerve (Gernot, 2016). Doctors are now trialling a device which stimulates the vagus nerve in arthritic patients which will reduce pain and combat the disease.

Memory

While the vagus nerve has a number of effects on the social aspects of our lives, its effect on learning is not fully understood. This much is certain: stimulating the vagus nerve does help in better learning and helps us consolidate the information we have just absorbed. This doesn't mean you'll turn into a learning machine like something out of the Matrix, but studies have shown that information consolidation does occur post vagal stimulation (Gernot, 2016).

One of the reasons for this effect is thought to be the release of the hormone norepinephrine into the amygdala. The amygdala sits at the base of the cerebral cortex and as we've seen, the vagus nerve connects directly into this portion of the brain. Norepinephrine helps increase memory retention and consolidation and with this, the stimulation of the vagus nerve helps memory.

Studies conducted on other mammals show the same effect as well. One particular study carried out in 2004 stands out. In this, researchers stimulated the vagus nerve of rats and found an increase in their ability to retain information, thus indicating higher levels of memory retention.

Emotional events help the formation of memories. What I mean to say is that the deeper the emotional impact of a particular event, be it positive or negative, the deeper it embeds itself into your memory. Scientists always knew this but could never quite figure out how norepinephrine was delivered to the amygdala. Well, thanks to this study, we now know that the vagus nerve is the answer. This is an extremely helpful find since it can help treat people suffering from PTSD and other memory related diseases.

There are implications for those suffering from Alzheimer's and dementia as well. Scientists have been trialing various drugs which regulate the level of hormones in a patient in order to influence memory.

However, vagal stimulation might be the answer for these diseases as well.

Respiration

Breathing has been known since ancient times to calm us down and help regulate our stress responses. Ancient eastern practices of meditation and yoga place a huge amount of importance on the technique of breathing. Research conducted in this century has shown that breathing deeply stimulates the vagus nerve and perhaps this is why deep breathing helps calm us down (Gershon, 1998).

Breathing deeply seems to result in the secretion of the hormone acetylcholine which acts as an indicator to the lungs to get them to expand and let more air in. Breathing deeply or even holding your breath for a few counts seems to elicit greater production of this hormone and as a result, our well-being increases.

It isn't just the production of this hormone that helps us. The vagus nerve in essence listens to the way you're breathing and regulates your heartbeat. As your lungs take in more air, it sends messages to the brain and in response regulates your heartbeat to match the amount of air you're ingesting. This is why in stressful situations you initially feel short of breath because your heart rate increases massively to deal with the stressful situation as well as the lack of air it demands.

Those who have practiced and explored the art of breathing better must have heard of a man named Wim Hof. This superman has endured seemingly hellish conditions, such as sitting outside in a snowstorm with just one layer of clothing, thanks to his breathing techniques. Breathing directly affects and stimulates the vagus nerve and thus, one can see the benefits of advanced stimulation.

As far as the biological process of respiration is concerned, the vagus nerve is pretty central to everything. It innervates the diaphragm as well as the larynx and pharynx. It is also connected to the heart as we've seen and damage to it will result in major respiratory problems.

Remember how the vagus nerve observes blood pressure? Well, deep breathing activates neurons that alert the vagus nerve about it becoming too high once you take a few deep breaths. This causes the nerve to communicate to the heart that it needs to slow down and hence, your heart rate lowers and you restore calm to yourself.

Heart Function

As you've seen thus far, the vagus nerve is responsible for regulating your heartbeat. However, its effects on the heart go far beyond that. Given that it monitors a number of bodily functions, and that these functions depend on a steady supply of blood pumped by the heart, the vagus nerve is pretty central to healthy heart function.

A study conducted recently shows that stimulation of the vagus nerve produces heart rate effects which helps combat a number of diseases (Porges, 2007). While stimulation can be used to treat epilepsy and depression, stimulation of the dorsal vagus circuit can be used to treat heart failure. This is a major find due to the fact that most people who suffer from heart disease tend to be advanced in age and might not be best suited for surgery.

Stimulating the vagus nerve is a non-invasive process. In addition to this, conditions such as vasovagal syncope, which is one of the main causes of a person fainting, begins with the vagus nerve. By regulating blood pressure and heartbeat, the vagus nerve plays an important role in maintaining a lot of functions associated with the heart. Currently there is a trial being conducted for a device which can stimulate the dorsal circuit and can revive a person from heart failure.

Relaxation

As we've already seen, the vagus nerve plays an important role in getting your body and mind to relax. The ventral branch is mainly responsible for bringing you into a state of increased willingness to socialize while the dorsal circuit is responsible for a shutdown which plays out differently depending on whether your ventral circuit is active or not. Since I've already covered how these mechanisms work, I'm not going to repeat all of that here.

Gut Health

Depression has been linked to gut health and a major reason for this is that the hormone serotonin is produced in the gut (Porges, 2007). Traditional drugs which are prescribed to treat depression suppress the absorption of serotonin and bring about changes in mood. While this treatment method has been in existence for a long time, new research shows that vagus nerve stimulation or VNS might be a better option for unipolar or bi polar depression.

This involves, much like every other VNS method, the placement of a tiny disk which pulses and stimulates the vagus nerve. Much like how it does with the heart, the vagus nerve monitors the health of your gut and signals the brain accordingly. The difference here is that while the heart can change the rate at which it beats to modulate blood pressure, there is no such tool for the mind or the gut.

The gut simply receives what you get and the brain interprets it as best as it can given its sensory inputs. Poor gut health can lead to the vagus nerve signaling a lack of serotonin being produced and this causes a feeling of sadness which will bloom into depression over a long term (Porges, 2007). I'm excessively simplifying a complex biological process here but this is what happens in essence.

The vagus nerve has even been referred to as a serotonin superhighway between the gut and the brain. A study conducted at McMaster University concluded thus (Rosenberg, 2019):

"The vagus nerve is the tenth cranial nerve and is the main afferent pathway connecting the gut to the brain. The vagus nerve can transmit signals to the brain resulting in a reduction in depressive behavior as evidenced by the long-term beneficial effects of electrical stimulation of the vagus in patients with intractable depression.

The vagus is the major neural connection between gut and brain, and we have previously shown that ingestion of beneficial bacteria modulates behaviour and brain neurochemistry via this pathway. Given the high levels of serotonin in the gut, we considered if gut-brain signaling, and specifically the vagal pathway, might contribute to the therapeutic effect of oral selective serotonin reuptake inhibitors." (SSRI)

SSRI here refers to the drugs that are usually prescribed to treat depression. The study itself was conducted to understand how they work since their effects are known but methods are not. It was posited that the vagus nerve was the one doing the major lifting while the drugs merely produced an environment in the gut which got the nerve to signal the brain appropriately.

This was partially proven to be true. While the full details of how SSRIs work might not be known, scientists have concluded that instead of undertaking drug treatments, certain patients might be better off with vagal stimulation.

However, this doesn't mean that every single type of anti depression medication should be sworn off. There is evidence that noradrenaline reuptake inhibitors or NRIs don't stimulate or involve the vagus nerve as much as SSRIs do and work differently. Either way, the brain to gut health connection has been identified as being extremely important and the vagus nerve is at the center of it all.

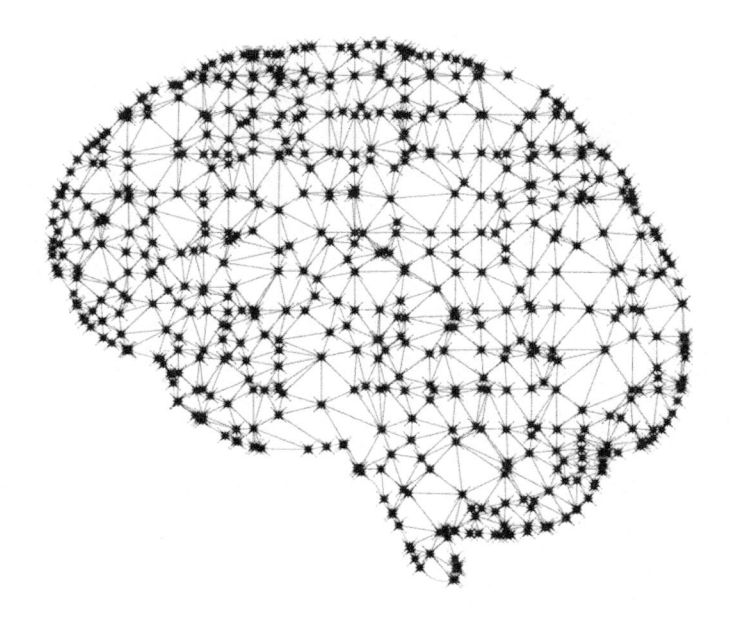

Response to Stress

I had mentioned the existence of a condition called vagal syncope previously. This is when a person faints thanks to a build up of stress and they simply lose consciousness. This often happens due to overstimulation of the vagus nerve. Generally speaking, any stressful situation demands a reaction from your heart and blood pressure.

The vagus nerve is at the center of it all and therefore is pretty crucial when it comes to regulating your response to stressful stimuli. An overstimulated vagus nerve will cause extreme reactions like the one described in the previous paragraph.

As you can see, there are many different functions the vagus nerve has. It affects almost every single major bodily function and this is why VNS is such an effective method of treatment for a variety of disorders.

Chapter 4: Diseases Associated With the Vagus Nerve and How to Prevent Them

The vagus nerve is sensitive to the factors that comprise your lifestyle. When it doesn't function properly, you are liable to suffer from a range of diseases and conditions. This chapter is going to walk you through the various diseases that occur due to the lack of function on the vagus nerve's part.

Do keep in mind that your vagus nerve is likely to malfunction equally due to lifestyle as well as certain congenital conditions. While the reasons for the malfunction may differ, the bottom line is that a healthy vagus nerve leads to a higher quality of life. So with that being said, let's look at the effects of the dorsal and ventral circuits on your overall health and well-being.

The Dorsal Vagal State

The dorsal circuit is often the cause of a number of issues. Since this is the initiator of the withdrawal reaction within us, it can take us down a positive or a negative path. As you've already learned, the difference between positive and negative really comes down to whether the ventral circuit is involved or not.

When faced with adverse conditions, two responses take place: The first is the activation of the fight or flight response and the other is the activation of the Dorsal vagal state. Under conditions of withdrawal our muscles lose their tension and go limp. This is accompanied by a feeling of exhaustion and heaviness. Recall if you've ever felt it a monumental task to simply move and pick something up. This is the dorsal state in a nutshell.

Other conditions that occur in a dorsal state include a feeling of flaccidity within your muscles, general tiredness, and lethargy. All of this is with your body. Mentally, a whole host of issues crop up. Feelings of helplessness, feeling apathetic and hopeless are the usual conditions our mind will experience in a pure dorsal state. A reason for this lack of happiness and the existence of lethargy is biological.

Remember that the dorsal state is one akin to hibernation. Your body is literally shutting down. Your heart rate lowers along with your blood pressure. Whatever blood is being pumped is moved towards the center of your body which leaves your limbs without a lot of oxygen to draw. The priority here is to enable basic internal functions and that's it. If your feelings of depression have been accompanied by the feeling of clamminess in your hands and feet, this is essentially what is happening.

Symptoms of fibromyalgia often occur in a dorsal vagal state. You will likely feel pains in your body. To be more precise, you will feel a pain that jumps around all over the place. Massage therapy is usually prescribed for such disorders but a therapist will be flummoxed by this type of pain. After loosening one tight muscle, the patient will complain of pain in another part of their body where nothing was wrong previously.

All of this ends up with the therapist chasing the pain without ever solving it. Of course, with our understanding of the vagus nerve, we now know that the solution to this conundrum is to activate the ventral circuit. I will discuss how exactly to do this in the latter half of this book.

Dizziness and Fainting

Vagal syncope has been mentioned before and is one of the most observable symptoms and conditions of a malfunctioning vagus nerve (Rosenberg, 2019). Please note that I use the word malfunction in the context of the ventral circuit not activating to alleviate the effects of the dorsal circuit. This lack of calibration or activation is the issue. Some people end up thinking that the entire dorsal circuit is at fault, and this is not the case.

Dizziness and fainting occurs due to low blood pressure. When your muscles lose their tonality, blood does not meet with much resistance and hence can flow through easily at lower pressures. Physical symptoms include sagging facial muscles and a loss of color in the face. Changes in vocal tone are a tell tale sign as well.

You will likely have issues modulating or changing your vocal tone and your voice will become flat. The eyes will also lose their sparkle, so to speak.

POTS

POTS stands for Postural Orth-static Tachycardia Syndrome. This is a fancy name for the condition when you feel dizzy if you stand up too fast. In some cases those who suffer from POTS may even faint if they stand up quickly. People suffering from this condition exhibit multiple symptoms of nervous system deregulation.

The nervous system is in charge of deciding how much blood goes where and the vagus nerve plays an important role in it. Thus, a malfunctioning or poorly calibrated dorsal circuit results in lower blood pressure and a lower heart rate which leads to a lack of blood flowing to the right areas when you change your posture.

A properly functioning nervous system makes the necessary changes to heart rate, vascular tone, and blood pressure when you stand up. Thanks to the system being imbalanced or poorly calibrated in those suffering from POTS, a lack of blood flow compensation happens. The net result is blood not reaching your brain and you end up fainting or feeling extremely dizzy.

Feelings of sweating and nausea which occur constantly also indicate an overactive dorsal circuit. Such reactions are common when we're faced with a life threatening situation. The problem is that there are very few such genuine situations in our world these days and the dorsal circuit treats everything a crisis. Bladder control also deteriorates and your breathing will slow down.

However, your breath will not be the deep and contented one of someone who is in a meditative state. Instead, your breath will turn shallow and the volume of air you inhale will be lower than usual. Since the dorsal state activates our survival instincts, you will experience a high level of awareness about what's going on inside you. Again, this is not the presence or awareness of a meditative state.

The meditative state is characterized by acceptance, whereas this state is more of fear and watching out for everything. Experiencing an out of body experience is normal under such circumstances. Perhaps a better way to describe this would be to say that you will feel a disconnect with yourself in such times.

Memory Loss

Wen in the dorsal state, blood flow to your brain reduces. This means you will have a hard time remembering things. Most people do not remember the events of the trauma they suffered from. This is because their brain literally shut down and did not record anything that was happening. They simply disconnected and viewed the whole thing as an out of body experience.

In such situations, the victim's brain literally descended down one step on the evolution ladder and reacted from a more primitive portion of itself. As such, their brain will lose the ability to verbalize or recall any visual information about the event. People with overactive dorsal circuits exhibit this sort of behavior as well.

While they might not exhibit the exact symptoms of someone who has undergone trauma, their memories will be hazy and will lack definition. As a result, they will find themselves being marginalized and this leads to problems which make things worse.

Depression and Anxiety

A lack of concrete memories or vocalization about certain events leads people to dissociate from life in general. This dissociation in turn further enforces the activity of the dorsal circuit which keeps us in a constant state of fear. I'm not saying someone will be shivering with fright but this manifests in regular activities.

Constant worry about everything is a sign of a psychological state of fear. A person with an overactive dorsal circuit will worry even when things are going well for them and their loved ones, objectively speaking. A lack of empathy for situations or for someone else is also a sign of this.

A lack of empathy often conjures images of cold heartedness, but that's not what I'm referring to here. The person suffering from an overactive dorsal circuit will be unable to look at anything beyond themselves and will hence remain in a state of constant worry when it comes to themselves and everyone around them. They may display a curious lack of concern towards those who are unconnected to them. Lack of empathy means not being able to place themselves in another's shoes. It should not be confused with exhibiting sympathy for someone else.

A lack of anything meaningful to contribute to conversations and saying a lot of words but communicating very little of substance is another result of this condition. This leads to an inability to form strong social connections and increases isolation. In addition to this, people with a poorly calibrated dorsal circuit will be unable to set concrete goals and take action towards them. It may seem from the outside that they're obviously in a bad situation or a poor one but their lack of action can be maddening to those who do not understand what is going on with them.

All of this only increases the state of depression within the person. If they used to function well, their current state and the helpless feeling it produces will give rise to high levels of anxiety within them.

All in all the dorsal state requires the intervention of the ventral circuit to help move a person from isolation to socialization. I'm not saying the ventral state is going to make you the life and soul of the party, but it will reduce the feelings of depression and anxiety that prolonged dorsal activity causes.

The Ventral State

As you've already learned the ventral state has everything to do with us adopting a more social attitude towards the things in our lives. This has the effect of modulating the dorsal circuit and turns the state of withdrawal into something that is far more conducive to developing intimacy and trust. In short, the ventral state provides a powerful push to us when it comes to enhancing the quality of our lives.

The ventral circuit is found only in mammals and in order to activate it, feelings of safety in the prevalent environment is crucial. The feeling of safety comes from what's going on within as well. Good health and a happy frame of mind are essential for proper functioning of the ventral circuit. Disease of any kind tends to shut this down since it is non essential for survival.

Sometimes, people mistake activity or mobility as being equivalent to an active ventral state, but this is not the case. Indeed, deeply dorsal states of immobility can be modulated with ventral states as well. While exercise and mobility does induce it, these are not the only things to do so. The best way to think of this is to view the ventral state as being one of social engagement.

The two state model depicts social engagement as being the opposite of stress and as a part of relaxation. However, social engagement in the polyvagal theory goes beyond simple relaxation. It is the very essence of our lives. Think of it this way: The dorsal vagal state is what we need to survive, but the ventral state is what enables us to truly live. One can survive with high levels of stress, but it isn't much of a life.

Social isolation leads to the ventral circuit being disabled and this state compounds the problem thanks to the dorsal circuit taking over, which only enhances the feelings of loneliness and depression. Once these feelings get bad enough, the sympathetic nervous system takes over and we enter a full fight or flight mode (Rosenberg, 2019).

As you can once again see, the functions of the dorsal and ventral circuits are very different, so why are these two clubbed together as being one whole 'vagus' nerve? Well, the fault largely lies with the ancient physicians who could not distinguish between the circuitry and functions of the two. They're not to blame for this because the cranial nerves are very intricate circuits and separating them is a tough task.

Also, one must take into account the complete lack of technology available back then. Galen, who was mentioned earlier as being one of the most prominent physicians of ancient Rome, has to sit around waiting for gladiatorial contests to explore the vagus nerve further. In between, he had to remain content with dissecting barbary apes and other animals like pigs to figure out basic anatomy. As such, we can excuse him this error.

The vagus nerve is better thought of as being a network. This network regulates a lot of your nervous system and is affected by your lifestyle. Once it is affected, the network in turn creates a set of conditions in your life which either makes things better or worse. Whether the ventral circuit is able to affect the dorsal circuit or not, decides the sort of situations you find yourself in.

As you can see, both circuits affect your levels of stress and anxiety. They don't directly cause it but both conditions are born thanks to the reactions of the autonomous nervous system. The vagus nerve/network plays a big part in determining how the nervous system proceeds to deal with a situation.

There are many afflictions that occur thanks to this and in fact, it is possible to connect your lifestyle and reactions to stress (your nervous system's conclusions) to a lot of diseases you might be currently experiencing. The ones highlighted in this chapter can be thought of as being direct results of a poorly calibrated vagus network. All in all, a healthy vagus nerve brings about a better quality of life. Of this, there is no doubt.

Let us now take a look at how stress and anxiety are born within the nervous system and the role the vagus nerve plays in the entire structure.

Chapter 5: Stress, Anxiety and the Vagus Nerve

Before getting into the details of depression and stress with regards to the nervous system, I'd like to clarify a few things. First, the usage of the words depression and stress is often wrong. For example, lifting weights at the gym puts your body under 'stress'. This is not a bad thing since it helps make you stronger. Similarly, being pushed to deliver work by a deadline is not bad 'stress'. It makes you more efficient.

We are constrained by language in such cases. Hence, to make it amply clear, when I refer to stress in this chapter or in this book, I'm referring to the activation of the sympathetic nervous system within us. This is the medically accepted usage and this is what I'll stick with moving forward.

The Sympathetic Nervous System

Stress was often thought of as being the opposite of relaxation. The fight or flight response was directly opposed to the state of bliss which was what relaxation was lumped under. As you've seen thus far, it's a bit more complicated than that. Polyvagal theory shows us that the vagus nerve induces both stress as well as relaxation depending on which circuit is active.

This doesn't quite fit neatly into the old model. After all, how is one to classify the dorsal circuit since it can induce both states? The two state model considered the vagus nerve as being responsible solely for relaxation and happiness and this isn't quite right. Stress in reality is the mobilization that occurs within the body in response to fear. This can happen due to stimuli from something external or internal.

Physically, this means our muscles are primed to make extraordinary efforts to take action to save our lives in this situation. As long as the threat is present, the sympathetic nervous system is in operation. Once the threat subsides, the problem begins as far as stress is concerned. In a healthy individual, the sympathetic nervous system should deactivate and the person should return to normal.

However, constant activation of the sympathetic nervous system creates a habit of sorts. Chronic activation can be a result of lifestyle factors and certain mental states. Things such as perfectionism, a lack of empathy and so on trigger mental states which are conducive for the sympathetic nervous system to kick in. Of course, once it kicks in, we're prone to evaluating pretty much everything in a binary threat/not a threat fashion and this results in even more stress being heaped upon us.

We create a vicious circle for ourselves in this manner. I must point out that the sympathetic nervous system isn't all bad. It does have vital roles to play. For example, in healthy individuals, the sympathetic system is called into action when we inhale. This increases our heart rate and blood pressure. With every exhale it is switched off again. Don't misunderstand this as you entering fight/flight with every inbreath. It's a bit more complicated than that.

Let's take a deeper look at what happens when the sympathetic nervous system or fight/flight is enabled within us.

Fight or Flight

Every animal on this planet has a fight response under stress. Reptiles are capable of significant feats of strength when placed in dangerous situations or ones which are essential for their survival. If a crocodile deems you tasty enough, it can run after you at half the speed of an Olympic sprinter if need be (Rosenberg, 2019). Similarly, snakes are equally capable of feats of physical strength which you wouldn't associate with them.

Within humans the fight state mobilizes a bunch of internal processes and organs to help us combat the situation. I've already detailed a lot of these so I'm not going to go over these all over again. Suffice it to say that in such a state you are primed to take action and your body is willing and able to assist you.

The old two state model confined the fight or flight response to the realm of stress. However, this is not the case. The sympathetic nervous can be deployed as a defensive strategy when not in a social situation. When in a social situation, it can actually boost performance. For example, prior to an athletic event or sporting task, the sympathetic nervous system can boost our body to provide us with that extra kick.

When flirting with someone, the sympathetic nervous system plays an important part in bridging the physical gap and initiating sexual foreplay. When the social aspect of us is not engaged, the sympathetic nervous system can express the fight within itself through a range of behaviors such as aggressive or proface speech towards someone. Sarcasm aimed at humiliating another person is also a manifestation of the fight response from the sympathetic nervous system. Other examples include passive aggressiveness, unjustified destruction of property (yours or someone else's), random aggressive behavior and so on.

In short, the fight aspect is misunderstood and is influenced by the social engagement aspect within us (the ventral circuit). Similarly, flight is equally misunderstood. It isn't just about running away from a situation. Flight could also mean a person avoiding a potentially troublesome situation entirely to escape potential hurt.

Troubled people who abuse drugs or seek unhealthy outlets are placing themselves in a state of flight when they consume these things. While drugs and alcohol are obvious examples, they aren't the only ones. A person constantly watching TV or sitting in front of a computer to kill time is also indulging in a flight responds to avoid anxiety that a social situation brings.

The Truth About Stress and Healing

Our brain's evolution holds a lot of lessons for the ways in which we need to approach dealing with stress and its effects. The entire autonomic nervous system can be boiled down to three different networks which operate on a hierarchical basis. Again, I'm simplifying a lot of things here but for the purposes of this book, this explanation is valid.

The first and latest in terms of evolution is the ventral circuit. As explained earlier, this circuit isn't found in too many mammals and promotes socialized immobility which enables us to relax and form stronger bonds. These bonds in turn help us deal with and reduce stress significantly in our lives as numerous studies have shown (Porges, 2007). Perhaps the very fact that this circuit has evolved points to our species adapting to our need for a higher quality of life than just mere survival. However, this is pure speculation at this point.

Next on the list comes our sympathetic nervous system which is what the fight or flight response is. The previous section covers all of this in detail and by now you must have a good idea of what this entails. The fight or flight response is present in pretty much every animal on this planet and under the old two state model, this was the 'negative' side of things.

Lastly, we have the dorsal circuit which is the least evolved and most common. It is the most primitive and in most animals, if the sympathetic nervous system fails to accomplish survival, withdrawal is deemed the best option and the dorsal circuit achieves this goal. As you can see, these three categories or systems range from being the most evolved to the least.

When a person mentions they're feeling stressed or are under stress, this merely refers to their emotions in the moment. From a biological sense they might not be in such a state. Stress is when people are in the second category and depression is merely the emotion a person feels when they're in the third category, when they've fully withdrawn and are in the dorsal state of mind.

Anxiety is a symptom of being in the clutches of the fight or flight mode (sympathetic nervous system). The interesting thing about these categories is that our brain moves through them in a progressive manner. If the ventral circuit is active, the other two lay dormant. Now, this doesn't mean they don't function but in terms of survival, they're not exerting themselves.

Thus, you could be in a highly sociable state but your sympathetic nervous system is exerting itself with regards to your breathing and your pulse. Your dorsal system is reading the signs for when withdrawal will present a good strategy for extended survival. When the ventral circuit switches off, you move directly into fight or flight mode as far as survival is concerned. When this fails, you withdraw.

Hopefully you can now see how your depression and anxiety develop. Thanks to the ventral circuit being completely inactive in proceedings, your nervous system kicks you into the more primitive circuits of your brain and in such a state, you desire a 'life', with its attendant pleasures, but your brain is in survival mode. In other modes you're prioritizing something but your nervous system is prioritizing something else entirely thanks to it being miscalibrated.

People can have the ventral circuits switched off thanks to prior trauma or certain triggers which place them in the grasp of their sympathetic nervous system for the majority of the time. This makes the activation of the fight or flight response a habit. The brain learns from its environment and whatever it does most often is what it will continue to do as time progresses (Porges, 2007). This, in essence, is what a habit is.

Activating the ventral branch is what short circuits this old habit pattern and puts us in a state which can be thought of as being 'advanced' survival. In other words, you're looking to live, not just survive. An active ventral branch lifts you from chronic activation of the sympathetic nervous system and the dorsal state.

While the determination of which state you need to be in is progressive when reacting to a stimulus, moving up the evolutionary scale is not so. In other words, you can move directly from the dorsal state to the ventral state via activation of the ventral circuit. While the ventral circuit is the ideal state, understand that engaging the sympathetic nervous system is a good option to move up from a dorsal state.

This is why competition and athletic activity beats depression. These activities simulate fight or flight situations and can help patients deal with lethargy and depression. In fact, most antidepressants work in this manner (Porges, 2007). They stress the body chemically by inhibiting certain hormones in our body and thus simulate conditions where it needs to now fight for survival.

No medication can ever stimulate the ventral circuit, though. Besides, when taking medication, one needs to deal with side effects as well which can be pretty unpleasant. All in all, exercises which activate the ventral circuit are a far better option when looking to lift yourself out of the dorsal (depressed) state.

The long and short of all this is that social engagement is the key to our well-being. Does this mean introverts are doomed? Well, not quite. Again, understand that I'm not asking you to go out there and be the center of attention and the life of every gathering. Every person has their own social thermostat. In other words, there is a different level for each person which marks them as being socially engaged and in communication with those around them. For some people this might mean being the center of attention. For others, it might mean sitting back and taking part in an engaging group discussion even if they aren't saying much.

Your emotional state and levels of relaxation are what indicate whether or not you're in this state. If you're in a situation where you're deeply uncomfortable and feel as if you have to say something, this is an indication of you being in the grasp of your sympathetic nervous system. Too much of this and you'll move into the dorsal state which will lead to depression.

The first step toward recovery is to determine whether or not your ventral circuit is active. Often, people have no idea how to do this and I'll show you how you can determine whether it is functioning or not. Once this is determined, you need to carry out the exercises described in the latter chapters of this book to help you move into a ventral state. This will automatically lift you from the dorsal or sympathetic state.

There are a range of techniques you can use to achieve this and you'll learn all about them. Most of all, you must understand that you can treat your depression and anxiety naturally and without medication. It is a tall claim but as you can see from all of the evidence and information I have placed before you thus far, it is completely possible to do so. The best part of this mode of treatment is that it doesn't matter whether you're taking your medication or not. It works nonetheless.

Treatment is really all about activating your ventral circuit and turning its activation into a habit. Once this happens, your brain will automatically start regulating its use and will be able to screen situations better. Thus, your brain will start working with you instead of against you. Understand that recovery is all a question of establishing the right habits, right down to the evolutionary level.

Most of us are simply unaware of how the vagus network works and thus, we end up relying on medication and a whole host of activities which move us from the dorsal state to the sympathetic level. We never realize that there is another level about that which makes things a whole lot easier. We might stumble onto this but turning its activation into a habit is where real improvement lies.

So now that you understand how stress and depression really come about, I'm sure you're keen on moving on to determining if your ventral circuit is working well. Before doing that, we need to take a small detour and revisit the polyvagal theory in more detail.

Chapter 6: Polyvagal Theory

Polyvagal theory fully explains the way our autonomous nervous system (ANS) really works. You will recall that the ANS was previously explained via the two state model which were named stress and relaxation. In biological circles, these were named sympathetic and parasympathetic. While not totally invalid, there are a lot of holes in this view of what is a very complex system.

Polyvagal theory posits that there aren't two but three levels or states to the ANS. I introduced this concept in the previous chapter where you learned about the three states the nervous system resides in. The most evolved state is the ventral state, followed by the sympathetic nervous system and then the dorsal state. This theory of our nervous system states that the vagus nerve is actually two completely different sets of circuits, with one overriding and influencing the other.

The two state theory considered the vagus nerve as being just one big nerve, and this is clearly incorrect. Such conclusions were brought about thanks to adhering to age old theories and from a failure to view the problem from different angles. Polyvagal theory changes all of that and helps us understand not only the nature of depression and anxiety better, but also their treatments.

The vagus nerve is at the center of polyvagal theory and we've looked at it in great detail this far. Let's now take a step back and consider the theory as a whole.

Thermostats

The best way to think of these three levels of the ANS is to liken them to a thermostat. The nerves in your body monitor your sensory responses and initiate the appropriate reaction. A good example of this is our physical reactions to our environment. When we feel cold, our body begins shivering. The muscle shivers produce additional heat. We can then place ourselves close to a source of heat or simply wear more layers of clothing to protect ourselves better.

The responses of our ANS can be hybrid as well. Hybrid here refers to a combination of two layers. Friendly competition is an example of a hybrid between the ventral circuit and the sympathetic nervous system. The result is a simulation of a fight or flight state but has none of the bad side effects. An expression of physical intimacy is a hybrid between the dorsal and ventral state as explained previously.

Together with the hybrid states, we have five states that the ANS operates in which is a far more flexible model of behavioral response as compared to the old relaxation versus stress model. Let's examine the ins and outs of the ANS a bit more and see how the cranial nerves play a role in all of this.

Neural Pathways

The first neural pathway, that is the ventral system, expresses itself through CN X (the vagus nerve) along with four other nerves, namely CN V, VII, IX and XI. This circuit promotes a soothing and relaxed feeling which makes us socially amiable and open. In addition to this, emotions such as joy, positivity, and love are associated with the ventral branch of the vagus nerve.

Behaviorally, it expresses itself through shared time and activities with friends, family, and loved ones. In evolutionary terms, cooperation increased our chances of survival and this is why social activity brings us a lot of positive emotions. Even introverts and loners (people who like being alone) need a basic level of social connection since this is hardwired into all of us, even if the degree to which we need this is different (Oschman, 2016). Talking, walking, singing, dancing together and so on are just expressions of this need as is making the decision to raise and nurture children.

The next neural pathway is the sympathetic nervous system as you know. This can also be referred to as the spinal sympathetic chain since most of the information with regards to this state is passed to the relevant organs via spinal nerves. This is when we heat ourselves up for movement, whether it be towards fighting or fleeing. Either way, survival is the ultimate aim here.

You can also think of this state resulting from your body being mobilized by fear. Emotions such as fear, anger, rage, and so on are associated with this neural pathway. When the sympathetic nervous system proves unequal to the task of dealing with the challenge we face, the dorsal system kicks in and this is the third neural pathway.

When faced with imminent destruction, our brain decides to immobilize us and chooses to conserve whatever energy is left. As I highlighted earlier, immobilization can be an effective survival tactic in nature when the odds are highly against a creature. In human beings the emotions of helplessness, apathy, and hopelessness are associated with this pathway. Physically speaking, your blood pressure drops, your muscles become loose and bodily functions realign themselves as described earlier. You might even faint or go into shock.

I highlighted the example of a mouse evading a hawk previously to illustrate how this can work, but a better example is that of an antelope or a gazelle escaping a lion in the wild. The fight or flight response kicks the antelope into action once it realizes it is being hunted. As it realizes the pride is overcoming it and that death is near, an antelope usually goes limp.

A lion is not a scavenger and as it's about to bite into its prey it realizes that the prey is dead already and this short circuits the lion's killer instinct. It does not eat dead things thanks to an evolutionary association with disease and death and hence drops its prey and moves on. Moments after this happens, the antelope rises back up and goes back to doing whatever it is antelopes do.

Similar suggestions have been made about avoiding tigers and bears, although the advice with regards to bears is iffy. Another good example of the dorsal circuit saving the day is when a porcupine rolls itself into a ball when a predator approaches, thus making it impossible for the predator to bite it (the porcupine) thanks to the quills sticking out.

There are two hybrid states as I mentioned earlier. The first hybrid state is when the ventral system combines with the sympathetic nervous system. This can be thought of as being a case of mobilization without fear. In this state the sympathetic system helps us mobilize our muscles and body in order to perform at our best while the ventral system ensures we remain on the right side of the rules and keep things within bounds.

It isn't just humans who play in this way. Puppies and dogs often play fight with one another and bark and growl at each other. However, there is no threat of harm implied in any of this. If you can be mobilized without fear, then you can be immobilized without it as well. This is when the dorsal state combines with the ventral state to produce a feeling of safety and intimacy. Lying down and cuddling with your partner is an example of this state.

The ultimate aim of the nervous system with all of these circuits is to maintain what is called homeostasis. Homeostasis refers to a state of dynamic equilibrium between a living organism and its environment. In other words, your reaction to your environment needs to be appropriate. Laughing at danger is a singularly un-homeostasis like behavior.

Neuroception

Neuroception was the term coined by Stephen Porges to describe the process by which neural circuits distinguish between safe and unsafe situations. The thing with neuroception is that it occurs outside of our conscious awareness (Oschman, 2016). In fact, it takes place in the deeply primitive portion of our brain and reacts automatically. Experiences of having a sixth sense and so on are examples of neuroception.

This doesn't mean our conscious mind doesn't pick up information. The decision making process is a complex interplay between the conscious and the subconscious portions of our brain. You can think of neuroception as being the processing of information that our conscious mind doesn't pick up. As such, it works a lot faster than conscious perception. How many times have you walked into a situation and just known something was wrong? Alternatively, how often have you started doing something and everything just felt right? This is neuroception in action.

As you can see, there is plenty of room for things to go wrong as well. If your neuroception is warped, then you'll end up categorizing a perfectly normal situation as being abnormal and everything you perceive will be colored by this initial thought. This is referred to as priming in psychological circles (Oschman, 2016). Priming can be thought of as defining the frame your mind is in. If you witness an act of kindness prior to walking into a tough negotiation, you're more likely to view the other side as being amicable to a win/win situation.

Priming explains why social media and the news tend to makes us feel miserable since all we see is hatred and stories of doom. When primed to believe the worst, you end up screening those very things into your life. Faulty neuroception can occur for a variety of reasons, ranging from deep seated trauma to short term priming.

You might be hungry and are hence cranky. Therefore you are less likely to put up with randomness in your activities. An example of deep seated trauma might be the way people react to dogs. There is evidence that human beings have effectively bred every single hostile fibre out of dogs to the point where dogs these days are compelled to be friendly towards everything except predators (Oschman, 2016).

Despite this, some people are scared of dogs thanks to childhood trauma. If a person was attacked by a dog as a child, they're likely to always believe that a charging dog wants to attack them. This is irrespective of whether the charging dog wants to play or attack. Neuroception ensures a faulty diagnosis of the situation. Generally speaking, neuroception is extremely open to manipulation.

Psychological triggers exist everywhere and some deep seated trigger might prejudice us in a given situation. We might be deeply in love with someone and we might not be able to see their flaws. We can literally be blinded by love, in other words. Chemical substances and medication can interfere with our neuroception as well. Antidepressants inhibit hormones and affect our perception of events as we've already seen.

It isn't just emotional matters that neuroception affects. Homeostatic perception is also affected. For example, some types of medication affect the brain's ability to detect cold. In such circumstances, you will not shiver and your body will not react to the cold until you suffer from hypothermia and die.

Trauma and Neuroception

Trauma plays an important role in the way we perceive things. Those who suffer from conditions such as PTSD have a tough time classifying things as being non-threatening and face huge challenges in managing their triggers. One of the reasons trauma is particularly challenging is due to the manner in which the brain learns and absorbs information.

The brain is a series of cells called neurons which are interconnected with one another to form what is called a neural network (Oschman, 2016). These networks together form a body of information. When sensory input is received, the connections fire up and a perception is formed. In turn the appropriate ANS pathway is activated to maintain homeostasis with the perceived environment.

The biggest weak link in all of this is neuroception. This is the filter through which we view the world and it is absurdly easy to manipulate as we've seen. Deeply emotional experiences, positive or negative, can color neuroception to the point where we turn facts on their head and become blind to everything else.

A good example of this is the standard of political debate. Political debate has never been of a high standard, contrary to popular perception. One reason for this is the need for people to cling onto their perception (neuroception) no matter what. Social media is one giant affirmation machine which only shows us the things we like to see. As a result, our biases build and the existing neural networks become stronger.

The brain is predisposed to minimizing the effort it must take to arrive at a decision. This is the goal of learning, after all. When you sit down to drive your car, you don't want your brain to go over the entire learning process all over again. You'd never reach anywhere if this happened. While this learning and reduction of effort is very helpful when it comes to driving, brushing your teeth, cooking your food and so on, it is actively harmful when it comes to neuroception which is colored by trauma.

Your brain simply reacts the way it always has and when you try to challenge this existing behavior, it simply rebels. After all, what is the need to do things differently? Remember that learning new things requires effort and this is also why we learn far less as we grow older when compared to children. We simply don't wish to make the effort.

It's a lot easier to cling onto what we already know and keep hammering it, even if we know it's wrong or not based on fact, since the alternative is just too much work. So what is the point of all this discussion? Well, for one thing, changing habits and beliefs requires you to apply an equal and opposite force.

In other words, you need to perform new behaviors and new mindsets with a high degree of positive emotion (why would you want to adopt a negative emotion on purpose after all?) and then repeat the action over and over. This is how learning takes place. Using the exercises I will highlight a few chapters from now, you can make the learning process easier for you since you'll be priming yourself for adopting new ways of thinking and improving your life.

All in all polyvagal theory will help you become more aware of which mental state you're in. This awareness alone is powerful enough to snap you out of your current mind and push you into another state. I'm not saying you should expect miracles. However, is change possible? It absolutely is!

Chapter 7: Testing Your Vagus Nerve

As you've learned by now, activating the ventral branch of your vagus nerve is what truly matters for your well-being. By activating this or by having a fully functional ventral branch, your ANS will kick into gear and assist you with your well-being. The first step to activating it is to figure out whether it is working or not.

Most people tend to have less than optimal ventral branches simply because we're not aware of their existence and do not use this with intent. What I mean to say is that your environment and lifestyle play important roles in ventral activation and without conscious effort on the health of your ventral branch, it can be easy to have it function at less than optimal levels.

In this chapter, you're going to learn all about evaluating your ventral branch's health. The last few chapters in this book, after this one, will deal exclusively with techniques you can employ to activate your ventral branch.

So let's dive right into it!

Basic Tests

The most basic test of ventral function is to evaluate whether someone is socially engaged or not in the majority of their conversations. This sounds simple enough, but a lot of human communication is non-verbal. So how does one evaluate this? The place to begin is the face. Facial muscles control pretty much everything to do with the amount of information you absorb.

This is because your nerves send sensory information back to your brain and depending on the kind of facial signals you're sending, your brain accordingly acts to maintain homeostasis. For example, if you're talking to someone and their eyes are closed, what does this indicate? Even better, have you ever tried participating in a conversation or tried to absorb information from a public setting with your eyes closed?

Some people find it valuable to close their eyes and concentrate on listening to something, but this is often when we need isolation. The point is that closing our eyes increases our isolation and hence decreases social function. When you're seated in a lecture hall, it is a brave soul who closes her eyes and then claims she was trying to listen to her professor with greater concentration instead of falling asleep.

The facial muscles around the eyes control the opening and closing of them. The ones above the eyes and between the eyebrows also control our reactions to events and indicate whether we're socially engaged or not. If someone tells you a piece of shocking news and you're distracted, your reaction to that piece of information begins with your facial muscles before you ever utter a word. We raise our eyebrows, narrow our eyes, widen them and so on to communicate a lot of things.

The muscles in our cheeks and lower portion of the face play an important role as well. When not saying anything, we stretch and manipulate the shape of our mouths to communicate. Tight facial muscles cannot communicate much beyond apathy to the situation. Thus, if you have tight muscles that feel as if they haven't moved in years, chances are your social engagement is low and as a result, your ventral circuit is not functioning optimally.

Beyond this, our facial muscles are also responsible for creating a number of faces which we use to communicate. All of these faces and their characteristics can be boiled down to three categories.

The Three Faces

The three faces are those we adopt unconsciously. These faces are your resting face, your face which reflects your current mood, and your face which reflects emotions directed towards someone else.

The third category is not an easily labeled one, so let's begin by looking at that. If you ever notice the faces of infants or children, you will see that their facial muscles change in tension rapidly and indicate a wide variety of emotions.

This behavior is not seen in adults very often, except in intimate romantic situations. In these situations, communication is fully open and there is no barrier to it between two people. Under such circumstances, we let our emotions flow without any censorship and this is reflected in our faces. As such, these kinds of twitches in our face indicate a state of openness and trust in the other person.

It is hard for the other person to read each and every twitch that occurs in such situations. However, from an evolutionary perspective, this sort of reading is unnecessary (Rosenberg, 2019). After all, if this behavior only occurs when a person fully trusts you and is being completely open with you, then what is the need to evaluate every single expression? Such a state also indicates a lack of fear with respect to the other person or the situation as a whole.

The second face we adopt is one which indicates our current mood. This face can last for as long as our mood exists and communicates to other people how we currently feel. Things such as our neuroception, speech, and so on are directly born out of this. The brain takes its cues from the face we make and accordingly aligns the appropriate system to take over.

Please note that you can have an active ventral circuit even in a situation when you're feeling annoyed. After all, it is social engagement that counts, not feelings of happiness or sadness. Sadness can be a bonding tool as well. For example, funerals have the potential of bringing estranged family members together and increasing their togetherness, especially if the person who passed away was a dearly loved one.

The first face that we pull is one of chronic stress. The quality of our lifestyle and mindset leaves marks on our face. The saying that a person more or less receives the face they deserve by the end of their lifetime is very true. Things such as wrinkles, the type of skin around our eyes, and so on reflect our well-being.

Either way, facial muscles are a huge indicator in the activity of the ventral circuit. You can examine yourself or ask someone you trust to make note of the faces you pull when in conversation or how your muscles twitch and react when interacting with someone. All of these are telltale signs of your quality of social engagement.

Vocal expression is directly related to facial activity. How often does you voice change pitch and tone? Do you communicate emotions with your voice? Or is it monotone and flat? The ANS affects your interactions with those around you. The fact is that while your personality has a base or a bedrock, your individual reactions to people depend greatly on the current state you're in.

If you're feeling like you need some alone time, your sentences will be short and curt. This might give the person you're interacting with the impression that you're rude or not a very accomodating type. If you had met them when you were in full ventral flow, the impression you would have made would have been very different.

One often sees depressed people sigh or breathe out before they talk. Their shoulders droop and their gait is labored. Their faces indicate no expression at all and their facial muscles might as well be hewn from rock. I'm not saying that people with poker faces are depressed. The point is that facial muscles provide an early clue as to what a person's current state is and whether their ventral circuit is operating at the time or not.

Physical and Emotional Malfunctions

There are different ways in which symptoms of ventral malfunction manifest. Broadly speaking, we can classify these as being:

1. Chronic physical symptoms
2. Emotional issues
3. Heart and lung issues
4. Bodily function disorders
5. Immunity issues
6. Behavioral problems
7. Mental issues
8. Miscellaneous problems

Let's look at these one by one.

Chronic Physical Symptoms

We've already seen how facial muscles provide an early clue as to how the ventral circuit is functioning. Generally, the tenseness or level of relaxation in a person's muscles is a good indicator of social engagement. If your muscles and body feel heavy and tight, then this is a telltale sign of ventral inactivity. Things such as migraines, clenching your teeth tightly or grinding them at night are also important signs you should take note of.

The feeling of having a lump in the throat, clammy hands, arthritis, and unjustified sweating are all signs of a malfunctioning or inactive ventral circuit in the moment. The longer or more chronic these symptoms are, the worse the activity of your ventral circuit is.

Emotional Issues

Being irritable or having a quick temper, crying easily, feeling lethargic, and so on are great indicators of a poorly functioning ventral circuit. In addition to this, things such as daydreaming excessively, having difficulty falling asleep, forgetting things, and feeling intense frustration are also signs that a person is not fully engaging with the world around them.

Heart and Lung Issues

Those who experience excessive dorsal activation or sympathetic nervous system activation will suffer from conditions such as asthma or shortness of breath. The heartbeat might also be irregular and will be accompanied by chest pains. Also, high blood pressure levels or hyperventilation are symptoms.

Bodily Function Disorders

Appetite levels, whether non-existent or levels that drive a person to overeat, indicate ventral function. Digestion also suffers thanks to excessive dorsal activation. The reasons for this have been described in detail already. Generally speaking, your gut and stomach are the first to malfunction when you move out of the ventral state.

Things such as hyperacidity and heartburn also occur frequently. Again, I'd like to point out that these are valid symptoms only if they're chronic. Eating spicy food and getting heartburn once isn't an indicator that you've moved out of the ventral circuit and that you need to find help.

Immunity Issues

Given the priority the dorsal system places on survival, you would think its constant activation will ensure we maintain a base level of health. However, it doesn't work this way. Activation of the states other than the hybrid ones and the ventral state means that a large amount of stress is being placed on our body and with digestion being sidelined, it isn't absorbing all the nutrients it needs.

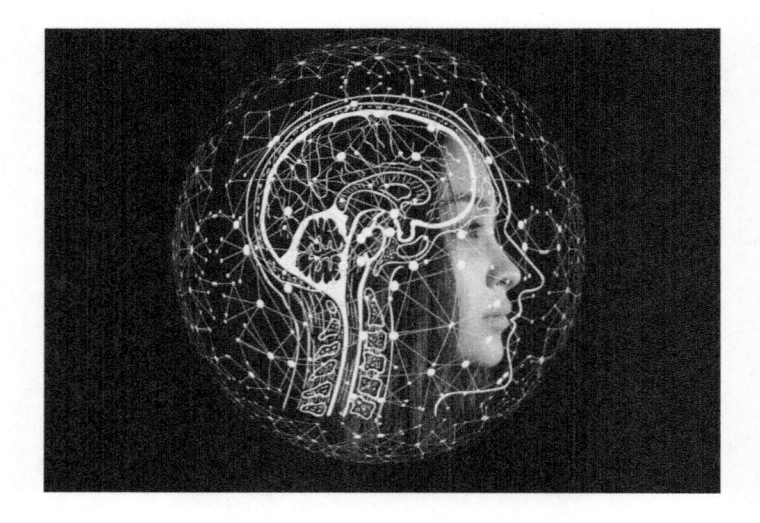

The net result is that the immune system suffers because it needs relaxation to fully arm itself. You will notice that people who are depressed tend to fall sick more often and when you feel down or low, you're liable to catch a cold or some small disease. Things like allergies and minor infections flare up all the time.

All of this is an indication that your ventral state isn't working well at that time.

Behavioral Problems

Substance abuse is a telltale sign of a lack of ventral activity. In addition to this, sudden mood changes, excessive smoking, and developing ADHD are signs of a lack of ventral activity. Getting into frequent minor accidents or sustaining injuries also indicate a lack of engagement with the world.

Mental Issues

Mental issues tend to poison our relationships by injecting a lack of trust into them. Things such as stubbornness and a lack of willingness in reaching accord with our partners, loss of sexual desire and so on indicate poor ventral activation. Again, these behaviors are an issue if they're chronic.

Such behavior is also accompanied by a lack of concentration, excessive worry and poor memory.

Miscellaneous Problems

Ventral circuit issues also manifest as contracting skin problems or experiencing excess menstrual pain in women. These miscellaneous issues indicate poor ventral health when combined with any of the other symptoms listed thus far.

Heart Rate Variability

Heart rate variability is an interesting field of research that has been gathering steam of late. When our nervous system is functioning well, our heart rate rises and falls according to the nature of our interaction, our hormone levels, and so on. I don't mean to say that your heart will be beating at 65 bpm one minute and 120 the next. That would be absurd.

Variability refers to much smaller differences. The thing to realize is that your heart rate will vary depending on the context of the situation you find yourself in. Scientists have concluded that a higher level of heart rate variability (HRV) is an indicator of good health (Rosenberg, 2019). When the ventral circuit is active, the HRV of a person tends to be high.

HRV is measured as being the difference in heart rate across specified intervals. These intervals can be fixed depending on the type of interaction you're having and the twists and turns that it takes. Generally speaking, the ventral state produces a far higher HRV than the dorsal or the sympathetic states.

There is also research that indicates a low HRV to psychological problems such as PTSD, emotional stress, and depression (Rosenberg, 2019). In addition, a low HRV also results in the inability to concentrate and in the occurrence of ADHD. There are numerous diseases and afflictions which are present along with a low HRV.

What is not known is whether the low HRV is the cause of this malfunction or whether it happens to be a secondary symptom. For example, a low HRV might be accompanied by depression. A depressed person is likely to turn to food to release their emotions and as a result is likely to become obese. So is obesity caused by a low HRV or is it the depression that is at fault? Generally speaking, obese people have been known to have low HRV rates but marking this as the cause of their obesity is a bit of a stretch at the moment (Rosenberg, 2019).

At the moment, we don't fully know how to increase HRV. All we know is that low ventral activity manifests in this condition. The preponderance of such findings leads us to believe that they are connected to the extent that HRV readings do indicate ventral activity. Whether it is directly caused by it is unknown.

There are further tests a licensed therapist or doctor can carry out. One of these medically oriented tests is to look at the state of what is called the Pharyngeal Ventral Branch function. This refers to the portion of the vagus network that innervates the throat. A doctor will be able to peer down your throat and look at the state of the Levator Veli Palatini muscles (Rosenberg, 2019). Dysfunction in the shape of these muscles indicates poor ventral function.

All in all, the best method of determining your own ventral function is to take a look at the list of behavioral and other chronic symptoms that have been listed in this chapter. A lot of them are caused directly by poor ventral function and are reliable indicators of this.

Chapter 8: Activating the Vagus Nerve

There are a few exercises you can perform to activate the ventral circuit for social engagement within yourself. Some of these you can perform all by yourself, while a few need the help of a licensed professional, usually a massage therapist or someone who comes recommended by a psychologist who understands the importance of the vagus nerve for our health.

This chapter and the following two are going to focus on nine different methods and techniques you can use to activate your ventral circuit. The first one is perhaps the most basic and easiest to perform. It also serves as a marker from where you can begin evaluating your vagal function.

So without further ado, let's look at this technique.

Basic Tracking

Before getting into the first exercise it helps to keep track of your symptoms prior to beginning the healing process. Given that the vagus nerve is entirely internal, it can be difficult to chart progress and map how much improvement you're experiencing. Look back at the list of symptoms and indicate how often they occur along with how severe they are.

You'll be doing this throughout your healing process and constantly noting the severity of your symptoms will help you figure out the progress you're making. It will also give you added motivation to do these exercises and seek help if need be. The first exercise we'll be looking at is termed the social engagement activation (SEA) exercise. Funnily enough, it doesn't require you to go out and start talking to people.

SEA aims to increase the level of mobility in the neck and spine by repositioning the C1 and C2 vertebra. This in turn increases blood flow to the brainstem and thus increases the function of the cranial nerves. Aside from the vagus nerve (CN X), it also helps the function of CN V, CN VII, CN IX and CN XI (Rosenberg, 2019).

All in all, this exercise takes less than a few minutes to complete.

S.E.A

Prior to beginning, twist your head to the right and note the freedom of movement you have. Hold that position for a few seconds and then bring it back to the center. Now twist it to the left as far as you can and bring it back to center. Did you feel any pain or stiffness when you did so? Note how far you were able to comfortably twist your head.

Once the exercise is done, you should perform this action again and note the improved mobility level. To begin the exercise, lie on your back. You can lie down on the floor or on your bed. Don't support your head with a pillow. Make sure the clothes you're wearing are comfortable and not excessively tight.

To support your head, interlock your fingers with one another and then place them below your head. This means your arms will be extended upwards and bent at the elbow as your head rests on your interlocked hands. Some people suffer from stiff shoulders so if you cannot lift both shoulders, balance your head with just one hand.

You should not press too hard onto your head with your fingers but neither should they be completely limp either. You should be able to feel your cranium with your fingers and the bones of your fingers in turn should be felt pretty easily on the back of your head. Make sure the entire surface of your palms makes contact with the side and back of your head.

Relax in this position for a few moments by taking a few deep breaths. Do not close your eyes since this is likely to result in your falling asleep. Keep your head centered through the exercise. Now, move your eyes to the right, and only your eyes. Do not turn your head to look right. Look as far to the right as possible for a period of thirty seconds to a minute. Usually, a period between thirty to forty seconds feels comfortable.

Keep looking to the right until you notice the following symptoms: swallowing, yawning, or sighing. Any of these mean that your autonomic nervous system is now relaxed. A sigh can be difficult to spot with the normal, relaxed breathing you're undertaking. A telltale sign of a sigh is when a shorter inhalation follows just before the exhalation, even if your initial inhalation has been deep.

Once you spot any of these signs, bring your eyes back to the center and look straight ahead. Now, turn your eyes to the left while keeping your head centered. Watch out for the same symptoms of ANS relaxation again. Once you spot any of them, bring your eyes back to the center and remove your hands from underneath your head. Remain in the lying down position for a few seconds and then slowly rise up. You might feel dizzy when you rise suddenly; this is normal. The reason this happens is due to the fact that your blood pressure was low during the relaxation exercise you just performed and standing up all of a sudden causes it to spike.

Once you stand up, move your neck to the right and left and check to see if mobility has increased. Also note any other changes in your overall physiology. How is your breathing? How do your muscles feel? And so on. Note any other feelings you have besides these, both physically and emotionally.

Why S.E.A Works

This exercise has physical reasons as to its effectiveness. Thanks to poor posture or emotional effects which cause poor posture in us, the spinal vertebrae C1 and C2 move out of alignment. As a result, increased pressure is placed on the vertebral artery which supplies blood to the frontal lobes of the brain and the brainstem. The nerves responsible for social engagement emanate from here, including the ventral vagus circuit.

There are patient and practitioner accounts of negative thoughts having the power to move these vertebrae out of alignment and cut off the social engagement functions, but these haven't been proved clinically as of yet. This much is clear, though: the spinal misalignment that takes place reduces blood flow to certain parts of the brain which enable us to function in a socially engaged manner.

There is evidence to suggest how this misalignment works. Ten muscles connect C1 and C2 to the occipital bone which exists at the base of the skull. Eight of these lie on the posterior or back of C1 and C2 whereas two lie on the front surface of the vertebrae. The occipital nerve innervates these muscles and hence any misalignment is immediately communicated to the brain.

What happens in essence is that the vertebral artery gets twisted and blood flow decreases. When you perform SEA and place your head in your palms, you end up stimulating the occipital nerve which relaxes the muscles and hence brings C1 and C2 into alignment. As a result, blood flows back into the brainstem and the nerves which control social engagement come alive once more. Hence, a lot of the symptoms of ventral deactivation disappear and relief steps in.

You might still be wondering why you need to move your eyes from side to side. Well, the eight suboccipital muscles and the muscles that move the eyeballs have a direct neurological connection. You can test this out for yourself. Place a finger at the base of your skull. This spot is somewhere near the top of your neck. Now roll your eyes up and down. You will feel a muscle twitch and stretch as you move your eyes. The upper cervical vertebrae moves along with our eyes, slightly, and the muscles change in tension as well.

The term misalignment with regards to the positioning of C1 and C2 can confuse people, so let me make this clear. The misalignment has biological purposes behind it, so it's not as if you're somehow malfunctioning if you find your C1 and C2 are not in alignment. Our thoughts influence the position of these vertebrae since the nerves that innervate them carry messages to and from them constantly.

C1 and C2 move out of alignment when we detect a threat in our environment and when the dorsal or sympathetic nervous state is required. This happens without our conscious knowledge and is a part of our survival mechanism. The only conscious thing you can do here is to bring them back into alignment to enable you to move into socially engaged states once more.

The point is that there is no fixed state in which you can maintain this alignment. Instead, balancing them is an ongoing process which you need to carry out whenever possible.

The Neuro Fascial Release Technique

This technique is a hands-on massage technique which was developed by Stanley Rosenberg using the principles of massage therapy, osteopathy, and anatomy (Rosenberg, 2019). It requires external assistance but is extremely beneficial in getting people to engage their social side. You can use it on yourself as well but when starting out, Rosenberg recommends having someone else do it on you.

He also recommends that this technique is better suited for children, infants, or those on the autism scale since it can be difficult to convey to the patient what they need to do. It is a basic technique and is hence an alternative to SEA.

Steps

Despite the hands-on nature of this technique, you will need to use your hands in a different way than in a normal massage. The aim of this exercise is to stimulate the nerves that lie under the skin just under the base of the skull. This helps balance any tension that exists in the muscles between the vertebrae and the base of the skull.

There is a one handed and two handed technique that can be used. The one handed technique begins with you laying the person on their stomach. You can do this with them sitting up as well but having them lie on their stomach enables you to see your hands better. Slide one palm of your hand onto the back of their head and feel the occipital bone at the base of their skull.

You want your touch to be light but not too light. As you feel the skin that covers the bone, slide it to the right and let it come back to neutral. Now slide to the left and let it spring back to neutral. Which direction did you encounter greater resistance in? Slid the skin back in that direction until you meet resistance.

The point here is to encounter resistance and gently relax at that point. You could encounter it less than half an inch to the right or left. Whatever the case is, slide the skin there and keep the light pressure on it. As you hold the skin in this position, you will hear the person yawn, sigh, or swallow. Much like in the previous exercise, this is a sign that the person's ANS is relaxed. If you feel for their C1 and C2 vertebrae, you will notice that they will be aligned.

If you don't know how to do this, don't worry, it isn't essential to the task. Keep monitoring the resistance or lack of it by sliding the skin to both sides. Hae the person twist their neck left and right to check their range of motion. You can have them do this prior to the exercise as well to set a benchmark.

Once you've carried out the one handed technique and mastered it, you can use the two handed version of this technique. This is a little more difficult to describe in words, but here goes. Have the person either sit or lie down on their stomach. Like in the one handed technique, test how easily the skin slides over the occipital bone. Usually, the skin will slide easily one direction as opposed to the other.

Hold the skin in this position and with your other hand, place a finger on the same side at the top of the neck. Push a little deeper with this finger and you will feel the muscles beneath. Slide the skin over these muscles and you will notice that they slide easily in the opposite direction to the skin being slid by your other hand.

Now lighten the pressure in both fingers and slide the skin towards one another in the direction of resistance. Stop once you feel resistance and maintain your position. Watch out for a sigh or a swallow from the person and once this happens, let go of your hold on them. Now do the same thing on the opposite side.

Once you perform this you will notice that the person will feel instant relief from a lot of what is bothering them. Of course, the ventral circuit can be switched off immediately as well thanks to the nature of their thoughts. The key is to regularly apply this technique for maximum benefit.

Technique

The key to making this technique work is to use as light a touch as possible. Traditional massage therapies have you placing a lot of pressure on the muscle and pushing the body inwards. This is not how you should be using your fingers here. You need to use the lightest touch possible. Rosenberg likens it to using a light touch where you can feel your skin melt into the other person's skin.

He mentions that if the other person can barely feel you doing anything, then this is excellent feedback. So take the time to understand how this technique works before putting it into practice.

Massages for Migraines

Migraines are extremely painful and when they occur, it is easy to lose all sense of balance with whatever it is you're doing in the moment. Migraines manifest differently for different people with varying triggers and pain points. The key to defeating migraines lies in applying the right sort of pressure to your trigger point.

These trigger points usually lie in the connective tissue between the skin and your bones. While your migraine pattern might be different, the trigger points are usually the same. Light massage of these points can reduce the pain significantly by activating your ventral circuit. Tension and hardness in these trigger points are responsible for migraine headaches.

These trigger points lie in a series from the base of your ear all the way down your neck to the trapezius muscle in your back, to where it meets the back shoulder. They exist on both sides of your neck and head. When suffering from a migraine or helping someone deal with it, run your hands down this chain and feel the muscle there.

You will notice that some points of this muscle feel tighter and harder than the rest. Massage these points and you'll be able to reduce the degree of pain significantly. The key to massage is to utilize the same technique as in the previous exercise. You don't want to push hard against the muscle. Instead, gently use your fingers to reduce tension. Hold the skin in the direction of greatest resistance and look out for a swallow or a sign which indicates ventral activity.

Once you spot this, move down the chain of trigger points and continue feeling for any tension. Slowly but surely, you will be able to bring relief. While you can choose to push hard against the trigger points, the fact is that this sort of force will flip the body into a dorsal state. A dorsal state will reduce the pain as well but without the interference from the ventral circuit, it isn't a desirable one to be in.

The body needs time to recover from a flip into the dorsal state. Instead, it is far better to apply light pressure and activate the ventral state so that the person can begin functioning immediately.

Chapter 9: Natural Ways of Activating the Vagus Nerve

Continuing our look at some of the ways to activate the ventral circuit of the vagus nerve, we're now going to look at the so called Salamander exercises. These exercises aim to increase flexibility in the spine and progress in difficulty. This doesn't mean you'll need massive strength to finish them.

It's just that the degree of flexibility they provide is greater as they progress. There are two levels to the exercises. Take your time understanding how they work and how you should go about performing them.

Let's now jump in and take a look at the first level of exercises.

Level One

The aim of all of the Salamander exercises is to free up the joints that exist between the ribs and the sternum. This directly affects your breathing capacity and your posture. These exercises will help reduce any forward tilt of your head and bring it back towards your spine. In addition, those who suffer from scoliosis or curvature of the spine will find these very useful in reducing this condition.

Before we get into the exercise though, I must note that eighty percent of the fibers of the vagus nerve are what are called afferent fibers. This means they are tasked with bringing information to the brain from the body. A small twenty percent are responsible for bringing information from the brain to the body. These are called efferent fibers. This is why physical exercises such as the ones in this chapter as well as the ones in the previous chapter are so effective.

By performing these, your vagus nerve is communicating to your brain that you are in a safe environment and that switching the dorsal network on isn't something that is going to maintain equilibrium. You could debate which affects which. For example, does shallow breathing limit ventral activity or is it the limited ventral activity which causes shallow breathing? This is a chicken or egg situation and there's no point delving into all of this for our purposes. At the end of the day, anything you do to alleviate your situation and activate ventral activity is going to help you.

With regards to the salamander exercises, a forward head posture limits the amount of air you can inhale. Furthermore, it also places a strain on the nerves which connect your head to your spinal cord. By fixing your posture, you can create more space for yourself in your upper chest and lungs. The reason these exercises are named this way is because you will maintain your head in a perfect line with your spine at all times, much like a salamander does. That creature doesn't have the ability to rotate its head independent of its spine.

During these exercises, your head position will be neither up nor down. The thoracic portion of your spine, that is the portion of your spine that corresponds to your chest area, will have greater freedom to move and you'll thus loosen the joints that exist in that portion of your body. This results in freer breathing and better blood flow through your chest. While the thoracic spine isn't designed for great flexibility in human beings, these exercises will result in above average flexibility in this area.

The Half Salamander

The first level of the salamander exercises comes in two parts. The first variation is as follows. Stand or sit upright as comfortably as you can. Take a few deep breaths. Once this is done, look to your right using just your eyeballs. Do not twist your neck to face that direction.

Now, while maintaining your gaze, bend your neck to the right until your right ear meets the top of your shoulder. Do not push the shoulder up to meet the ear. Hold this position for thirty seconds to a minute. Now do the same for the left side. You can repeat this exercise twice for each side.

The second variation of this exercise is when you gaze in the opposite direction to the one you've tilting your head in. So you begin by looking to the right and then tilting your head to the left until your left ear touches the left shoulder, or gets as close to it as possible. Then, bring your head back up and your gaze to the center.

Now, move your gaze to the left and bend your head so that your right ear is as close as possible to or is touching your right shoulder. Bring your head back up after holding the position for close to minute and bring your gaze back to the center.

Level Two

The next level is when you will perform the full salamander exercise. In this exercise you will move your entire spine instead of just your neck. To prepare, get down on all fours with your knees supporting yourself along with your palms. You can rest your palms on a cushion if this helps.

The thing to look out for in this level is that your head needs to be on the same level with your spine. Finding this exact point is difficult, so move your head up and down until you sense it is above or below your spine. Keep reducing the up and down movements of your head until you manage to locate the approximate level where your head is neutral. You could ask someone to spot you as well. Your ears should be on the same level as your spine. This is what indicates a neutral position.

Once you've found this level, look at the right. Next, bend your head, at the neck, towards your right shoulder. Allow this bend to flow down your torso as your spine curves in that direction as well. You don't need to pretend to be a snake; curve your spine towards the right as much as possible.

Now, release the curve and come back to the neutral position. Bring your gaze back to the middle. Now, look to the left and curve your spine in that direction like you just did. Hold your position for close to a minute and breathe normally throughout the process.

Releasing a Stiff Neck

While you're on your fours, you might as well perform an exercise which will release your stiff neck. This exercise will help relieve headaches and go a long way towards preventing migraines from occurring. The idea is to replicate the pose we adopted as infants where we laid on the floor and rested our weight on our hands and elbows and arched upwards so we could look around.

To begin, lie on your stomach with your arms out in front of you. don't extend them but just place them in front with your elbows perpendicular to your torso. Now, bring your chest up as much as possible and rotate your head to the right as much as you can. Hold this position for around a minute and bring your head back to center.

Now rotate your head to the left and hold it there for a minute. Generally, this exercise reduces the occurrence of a stiff neck unless there is a more serious injury you have sustained.

Natural Lifestyle Methods

Activating your vagus nerve isn't just a question of performing a few exercises. Perhaps the biggest thing you can do to help yourself is to lead a lifestyle that supports healthy activation of the ventral circuit. There are a number of things you can do, so let us take a look at these one by one.

Cold Therapy

Cold therapy has a number of benefits, but perhaps one of its best outcomes is the stimulation of the ventral circuit. This doesn't mean you apply an ice pack whenever you feel disturbed but if you find your body temperature increasing or if your heart rate is quickening, then applying an ice pack on your skin will help calm you down.

The reason for this is that a fast heart rate results in higher blood pressure. Tightness in your muscles increases and all of this communicates to your brain that it needs to push you into a fight or flight response or into a dorsal state. The ice pack or something equivalent lowers your body's temperature and also your heart rate, thereby communicating that everything is fine and that there's no need to panic.

This results in the ventral circuit being activated. Mind you, it's not going to turn itself on immediately, but it will help move you into a situation where you're a lot calmer and more conducive to having it activated within you.

Deep Breathing

The exercises I have listed thus far have included the act of breathing deeply at first. Deep breathing, as I've mentioned in this book previously, has been recognized since ancient times as being a key factor in our well-being. Deep breathing lowers our heart rate, causes us to expand our lungs, and simply communicates to our brain that there is no need to mobilize our emergency resources at this moment.

This automatically removes the sympathetic nervous system from the game. Now, you could move into the dorsal state without having your ventral state activated, so it is important that you accompany this with some form of exercise detailed previously. The same applies to cold therapy as well.

Moving Your Mouth and Using Your Vocal Chords

Chewing, singing, humming, and so on activate the ventral circuit of the vagus network. Chewing activates the digestive system and this is a direct signal to the brain that everything is fine. After all, you're not going to be chewing something when a lion is staring at you hungrily. Singing and humming also have the same effect since the vocal chords and the throat are innervated by the cranial nerves as you learned earlier in this book.

You don't need to swallow anything either. Chewing gum can help start the digestive process in which the vagus nerve plays an important role and will help calm you down.

Intermittent Fasting

This is a counterintuitive thing but intermittent fasting actually stimulates the ventral network. Generally speaking, fasting of any sort leads the body to conserve energy and move into a dorsal state, but intermittent fasting falls short of this. While it is a stretch to claim that intermittent fasting directly stimulates the vagus network, it does have immense health benefits.

These benefits in turn just put us in a better state to have the ventral network stimulated and allows it to shine, so to speak. The point is that getting healthy is always a good thing.

Probiotics and Clean Diets

This is a no brainer, not just for vagal stimulation but for good health overall. Your gut is directly connected to your brain thanks to the vagus nerve, and ensuring gut health goes a long way towards maintaining a positive and uplifting state of mind. The issue these days is that a lot of chemically processed food ends up killing the gut flora that ensure proper digestion.

Without the good bacteria in your gut which break down the food you eat, indigestion, leaky gut, irritable bowel syndrome and all sorts of disorders arise. Probiotics nurture gut flora and help you alleviate these conditions. Fermented foods such as kimchi and sauerkraut are great probiotic foods, as are Greek yogurts.

Beware of food that has added probiotics. There are many items on the market which are marketed as 'Greek style' and so on but in reality these are regularly produced food that has a few bacterial cultures added to them. There's not much evidence that these foods can replicate the action of a genuine probiotic.

Eating whole foods and a balanced diet goes a long way towards maintaining gut health. By balanced I mean even junk food. Junk food provides a release for our taste buds since they usually taste good and are addictive. The key is to consume small quantities of them. Junk food contains a doubly negative shot of both sugar and chemicals. Things such as monosodium glutamate (MSG) and high fructose corn syrup are used as preservatives, and you should stay away from these.

There are many diets out there but to be frank, you should simply focus on eating whole food for your meals. This means you need to cook your own food and consume food that is as close to its natural form as possible. Save the junk food for a cheat meal on the weekends. A lot of people complain that healthy food is tasteless. It's not the food that's the problem but your taste buds.

Having eaten processed sugar for so long, they're used to unnatural levels of sweetness. After consuming large quantities of processed sugar, the natural sweetness of fruits will seem bland. Give your taste buds time to adjust and they'll start to recognize the flavors in food again.

Fats and Omega-3

Here's the deal: Fat does not make you fat (Rosenberg, 2019). If there's one thing you need to take from this book (aside from ventral versus dorsal circuits), it is this. Healthy fats such as those present in dairy, butter, cheese and so on are good for you. You should ensure that you don't overdo it, that's all. So don't feel guilty about adding some cream to your sauces, it's fine as long as you don't overindulge.

Omega-3 is one of those superfoods and is found most frequently in fatty fish such as cod and mackerel. Sardines are a great little fish which are an excellent source of protein and omega-3. There are some supplements on the market which are marketed as omega-3 but whose oil is extracted from vegetables. Vegetable oil is not rich in omega-3 and as such, I recommend sticking to fish oil for this.

Cooking oil such as cold pressed olive oil and coconut oil is the best. Avoid highly processed oil such as canola or frying oils. The lighter the color of the oil is, the more chemicals it has gone through. Stick to cold pressed oils for cooking and you'll be fine. The best part of cold pressed oils is that they double as beauty products as well. Coconut oil is excellent for your hair and for moisturizing your skin. Olive oil also acts as a conditioner for your hair and so on.

Variety

This one is harder to pin down, but much like how your diet needs to be balanced, so does your life. It's fine to work hard, but make sure to avoid working at the expense of everything else. No matter what Elon Musk thinks, working all the time is not a good recipe for success or good health.

Incorporate exercise, socializing time, and boredom into your routine. Yes, boredom is good for you (Rosenberg, 2019). It allows you to recharge and brainstorm things to do which enhances your creativity. Instead of seeking to be entertained by your phone every second, put it down and just be bored. You'd be amazed at how many ideas come floating into your head.

Chapter 10: Other Simple Exercises to Activate the Vagus Nerve

This chapter is going to give you three more techniques you can use to activate your vagus nerve. The techniques in this chapter are pretty simple and also involve some ancient medicinal processes which activate the vagus nerve. The first is an exercise you can perform pretty much anywhere, so let's look at this first.

Twisting the Trapezius

The trapezius muscle is something all of use extensively when we're babies. When babies crawl around, they use all points of the trapezius to support their weight on their shoulder blades, lift themselves, and move forward. Once babies learn to walk, the trapezius is used unevenly and as a result imbalances develop.

A lot of us spend our days sitting in front of a computer and this causes us to lose our posture. Our shoulders roll forward and our bacs slouch. None of this is good for our long term posture and it results in imbalances in the joints and muscles in the back which leads to a lack of blood flow to our brain. As you can imagine this results in the ventral circuit receiving less than its share of blood.

The exercises I will highlight should ideally be done multiple times during the day to revitalize yourself and to readjust your posture to prevent it from going bad. Those who suffer from their heads leaning forward will also benefit from this. The result of carrying out these exercises is usually instant revitalization and energy. You won't start doing jumping jacks, but your energy levels will be higher than what they just were, that's for sure.

Steps

There are three ways of performing this exercise, so you can choose whichever one suits you the best. Ideally you should perform all three of them. To begin, sit on a comfortable surface or stand if that feels better. Take a few deep breaths and keep your eyes open. Now, bring your arms out in front of you and cross them. Let your palms rest on top of your elbows.

With your face looking forward, twist your torso towards one side. Don't think of this as twisting from the hips. Instead, move your elbows out to one side and then to the other, briskly. Do not stop in these movements or rest in between. Keep the moves brisk and twist thrice on either side. This activates the trapezius muscle fibers.

The second way or performing this is pretty much the same as the first, but instead of crossing your arms in front of you, cross them and hold them higher than your chest. Now twist from side to side while keeping your face as forward facing as possible. Remember to not rotate from the hips. Keep your hips stationary and only move your elbows from side to side.

The third way has you raising your arms above your head while still being crossed. Twist from side to side thrice and keep the movement brisk. Do not stop in between. Once the exercise is complete you will feel your head becoming lighter and moving back in line with your spine. You might feel taller thanks to this.

Acupuncture Techniques

Acupuncture has been shown to stimulate the vagus nerve effectively. The technique relies on stimulating certain points throughout the body. The techniques I will be highlighting here have to do with stimulating the facial muscles. Remember, the vagus nerve innervates portions of your face along with other cranial nerves, namely

CN V and CN VII. These techniques have the following benefits:

- Improves blood circulation in your face
- Makes your skin look fresh and vibrant
- Refreshes the corners of your eyes and mouth
- Relaxes the muscles that help you smile
- Loosens up the muscles in your face and opens you to deliver more expressions in social interactions

When performing this technique, look into a mirror. Perform them on one side of the face before moving on to the other side. You will notice your muscles relaxing on one side when you're finished with it.

Steps

The preliminary step for you to take is to find what is called the LI 20 point on your face. This is an acupuncture point and is where the endpoint of the large intestine is. No, your large intestine does not run up to your face. This is simply the meridian of the large intestine and it exists on this axis which happens to end on your face. In addition to this, the spot also lies directly over a joint between two bones. These bones are together referred to as the Maxilla but in infants, they used to be two, namely the pre-maxilla and the maxilla.

This spot is referred to as the beauty triangle in acupuncture and other eastern forms of massage. The spot lies about an eighth of an inch to the side, above the fold between the cheek and the upper lip. This point is usually more sensitive to touch with your finger so take the time to explore this area. Alternatively, you can refer to an acupuncture chart to get a fair idea of where this spot is.

With a finger, lightly brush the area. Apply pressure but so little that you can barely detect it. Your fingertip and the skin underneath should seem fused together. Slide the skin over this point up and down and note which direction provides greater resistance. Move the skin in that direction and hold it there until it releases. Now move the skin from side to side and again note which direction provides the greatest resistance.

Hold the skin against on that side until it gives way. Remember to keep your pressure light. This is not a massage. Now, increase your pressure ever so slightly. The objective is to stimulate the first layer of muscles underneath the skin. Once you become better at this technique, you will be able to feel the first layer moving against the second layer.

Move your finger around in circles and feel which direction has the greater resistance to it. Hold your finger in that direction for a short while until it gives way. Keep circling the spot until you feel almost no resistance. Now, increase your pressure until you can feel the bone underneath the skin.

Move your finger up and down and side to side and feel for increased resistance. Hold your finger in that direction until it releases. Remember to keep your push firm but not hard. You should feel the bone but don't press down hard on it.

You will find that the muscles around the corners of your mouth will relax immensely and you'll be able to smile a lot wider than previously. This is because the cranial nerves V and VII have been stimulated along with the vagus nerve. Over time, you will notice wrinkles decreasing as well. Relaxing the muscles underneath your face will give you a friendly and more gentle demeanor.

All of this will contribute towards your social engagement and you'll find your interactions becoming more pleasant.

Technique #2

The second technique works in the same way as the first but its focal point is different. In this exercise you will be focusing on the area around your eyes. This is referred to as acupuncture point B2 and it exists on the inside of your eyes, just in the area between your eyes and the top of your nose. Most of us rub this area when we're stressed naturally. If you're having problems finding this spot, you can refer to an acupuncture chart.

The muscles here are very thin and for this reason, it is best to use your thumb. Again, you want to feel the skin, then the muscle underneath and then the bone. The technique is the same. Begin by lightly running your thumb from side to side and look for the direction of greater resistance and lightly push against that until you spot a release.

Then move it up and down and look for a release in the direction where the greater resistance lies. Once this is done, press harder until you can feel the bone and move the skin up and down and side to side, looking for a release in the direction which offers the greatest resistance. Remember that while your press should be firm, you don't want to be pressing as hard as you would during a massage.

This pressure point directly stimulates the thin muscle that surrounds the eye called the orbicularis oculi. This control the opening and shutting of the eye and if imbalanced, your eye might be open too wide or simply not enough. The massage balances it out. In addition, massage also stimulates the lacrimal bone which plays a role in producing tears within the eye. While you don't need to be crying buckets, some level of moisture in your eyes gives them the twinkling look that is particularly alluring to others.

The goal of both the massages or facelifts if you will is to leave you looking refreshed and to present your best face to those around you. This will improve your social engagement and you will automatically stimulate your ventral circuit further.

When carrying out these actions you might feel as if you aren't doing too much, but resist the thought. The fact is that you don't need massive or forceful stimulation to engage the vagus nerve. The exercises also seem simple at first but the longer you perform them, the better your quality of life will be. Ultimately, this is a marker of how well you are stimulating your ventral circuit.

Conclusion

The pharmaceutical industry makes billions per year on drugs to combat depression, anxiety, and other lifestyle based disorders. While these drugs work to a certain extent, you will have to deal with the side effects that they produce. When seeking a chemical solution, there is no such thing as a free lunch. You need to balance the good with the bad and simply choose the option that produces the least worst outcome for you.

Given the complicated nature of how medicines work, vagus nerve stimulation can appear to be too simplistic at first. You might think that all you're doing is twisting this way and that and massaging this and that. How can such small actions bring about massive results? The pharmaceutical industry will tell you that all of this doesn't work and that depression is a chemical reaction that ought to be solved chemically.

Well, the thing about treating depression is that your aim is to try to get back to who you really are. In other words, you need to get back to your best self. Depression, anxiety, and other disorders such as these occur due to imbalances that are a product of our lifestyles. Bringing things back into balance is the ultimate aim. Drugs and medications do not achieve this since they always leave some chemical residue which causes side effects. Please note when I'm using the word drugs, I'm referring to prescribed ones as your doctor recommends. I'm not referring to narcotics or other escapes like them.

The vagus nerve, as you've learned, has been talked about for many centuries now. The truth is that we have everything we need to live a great life. It's just that as science has progressed, we've lost the balance between trusting ourselves and looking outward for a solution. Anything that doesn't seem complicated is dismissed too soon. Understand that the functions of the vagus nerve are extremely complex. It's just that, in this book, I've presented it in simple words for you to understand the power of this wonderful part of you.

While the vagus nerve is referred to as a

singular thing, it consists of two different neurological circuits, the dorsal and ventral. While the ventral circuit is the real difference maker in more evolved beings and enables us to live a high quality of life, don't be quick to dismiss the dorsal circuit. Given that it results in withdrawal, we might be tempted to think of it as being a retreat of sorts which offends our sense of bravery. The fact is, and I've given you multiple examples of this, withdrawal has deep biological roots and is a very effective tactic.

The issue for human beings is that we need a balance between ventral and dorsal activity to keep things functioning in our lives. Our default states, in the absence of ventral activity, are either the sympathetic nervous system which is the fight or flight response or the dorsal circuit which results in us withdrawing from life in general. Depression is a sign of dorsal activity without ventral intervention. Anxiety is simply the sympathetic nervous system creating nightmares for itself.

Your lifestyle plays a huge role in all of this. You can do all the exercises you want but unless you fix your lifestyle, all will be for naught. Things such as the level of exercise you perform, the quality of food you eat, and the degree to which you inhibit intake of substances which damage your health over the long run decide how active your ventral circuit is going to be.

The exercises themselves simply place you in a better spot to be recognized as someone who is socially engaged. Remember that the majority of human communication is non verbal. Therefore, the reactions of people around you have taken place long before they ever open their mouths and say something to you. By opening up and having the qualities of someone who is engaged, you will welcome social attention and automatically activate your ventral circuit.

If you're suffering from a deep depression you might ask how long this will take to give you results. Well, I wouldn't think of this in terms of hard results. It is your lifestyle, after all, that is being affected, and quantifying that is a slippery slope. My advice is that if vagal nerve stimulation is not working for you, or if you find yourself unable to bear the load that depression is placing on you, seek professional help immediately. Sharing the burden with a licensed professional will help you progress at a much faster rate and you will see changes quickly instead of suffering in silence within yourself.

The vagus nerve is a part of your body's function when it comes to creating a great life for itself. Stimulating it is a combination of using ancient techniques as well as utilizing modern research. It innervates pretty much everything in our body and you should always pay attention to your state if you're interested in living a high quality life.

I'm positive this book has given you everything you need to live a better life. Take the time to understand the science and the art of vagal stimulation. Let me know what you think of all of this and remember, you are not alone in your problems. Seek help and always keep in mind that you have everything you need to overcome your issues. I wish you all the luck and happiness in the world!

References

Carney, R., Freedland, K., & Veith, R. (2005). Depression, the Autonomic Nervous System, and Coronary Heart Disease. Psychosomatic Medicine, 67, S29-S33. doi: 10.1097/01.psy.0000162254.61556.d5

Gehin, A. (2007). Atlas of manipulative techniques for the cranium & face. Seattle, Wash.: Eastland Press.

Gernot, E. (2016). Heart rate variability. [Place of publication not identified]: Springer London Ltd.

Gershon, M. (1998). The second brain. New York: HarperCollinsPublishers.

Oschman, J. (2016). Energy medicine. Edinburgh: Elsevier.

Porges, S. (2007). The polyvagal perspective. Biological Psychology, 74(2), 116-143. doi: 10.1016/j.biopsycho.2006.06.009

Rosenberg, S. (2019). Accessing The Healing Power Of The Vagus Nerve. [S.L.]: Readhowyouwant Com Ltd.